MW01145119

SEE PAGE 128 FOR ORDERING INFORMATION

ABBREVIATIONS		h	hour	meq	milliequiv	PR	by rectum
bid	twice per day	Hb	hemoglobin	min	minute	prn	as needed
BP	blood pressure	HR	heart rate	ml	milliliters	qd	every day
cm	centimeters	ICP	intracranial	mo	month	qid	4 times/day
CNS	central nervous sys		pressure	NS	normal	SC	subcutaneous
CSF	cerebrospinal fluid	IM	intramuscular		saline	SD	standard
d	day	IO	intraosseous	O_2	oxygen		deviation
D_5W	5% dextrose in H_2O	IV	intravenous	PMN	neutrophil	SL	sublingual
ET	endotracheal	J	joules	PO	by mouth	tid	3 times/day
F	French	kg	kilograms	PPV	+pressure	µg	micrograms
g	grams	m^2	square meters		ventilation	yo	years old

Tarascon Publishing, Box 1522, Loma Linda, California 92354

Important Caution - Please Read This!

The information in *Emergency Medicine Pocketbook* is compiled from sources believed to be reliable, and exhaustive. Efforts have been put forth to make the book as accurate as possible. *However the accuracy and completeness of this work cannot be guaranteed.* Despite our best efforts this book may contain typographical errors and omissions. The *Emergency Medicine Pocketbook* is intended as a quick and convenient reminder of information you have already learned elsewhere. The contents are to be used as a guide only, and health care professionals should use sound clinical judgment and individualize therapy to each specific patient care situation. This book is not meant to be a replacement for training, experience, continuing medical education, or studying the latest drug prescribing literature. This book is sold without warranties of any kind, express or implied, and the publisher and author disclaim any liability, loss, or damage caused by the contents. *If you do not wish to be bound by the foregoing cautions & conditions, you may return your undamaged book for a full refund.*

The Adult Emergency Medicine Pocketbook

ISBN 1-882742-10-9. Copyright © 1999 Mako Publishing, Winter Park, Florida. Printed in the USA. All rights reserved. Published & marketed under exclusive license by Tarascon Publishing, a division of Tarascon Inc, Loma Linda, California. No portion of this publication may be reproduced or stored in a retrieval system in any form or by any means (including electronic, mechanical, photocopying, etc.) without prior written permission. The cover is a detail "Wound Man" indicating injuries from various weapons, by Parcelsus, Switzerland, 1536.

Universal Algorithm for Cardiac Arrest

Assess responsiveness

Responsive
- Observe
- Treat as indicated

Not Responsive
- Call code team or activate EMS
- Call for defibrillator
- Assess breathing

Breathing
- Maintain open airway

Not breathing
- Open airway, give 2 slow breaths
- Assess circulation

Pulse present

No pulse

- Rescue breathing
- Oxygen
- Start IV
- Vital signs
- Endotracheal intubation
- History
- Physical examination
- Monitor, EKG

Start CPR

Treat Suspected Cause
- Hypotension/shock/pulm edema
- Acute MI (page 17-19)
- Arrhythmia (page 11,13-15)

Ventricular fibrillation/tachycardia (VF/VT) present on monitor ?

No

Yes

- Endotracheal intubation
- Confirm tube placement
- Confirm ventilations
- Determine rhythm and cause

VF/VT
page 4

Electrical activity?

Yes

No

Pulseless electrical activity
Go to PEA page 5

Asystole
Go to page 5

Ventricular Fibrillation/Pulseless Ventricular Tachycardia (VF/VT)

- **ABCs**
- Perform **CPR** until defibrillator attached and consider precordial thump
- If **VF/VT** is present on monitor

↓

Defibrillate up to 3 times for persistent **VF/VT** if needed (200,300,360 Joules)

↓

Rhythm after defibrillation?

↓ ↓ ↓ ↓

| Persistent or recurrent VF or VT | Return of spontaneous circulation | PEA See page 5 | Asystole See page 5 |

↓ ↓

| Continue CPR · Intubate · IV access | · Assess vital signs · Support airway and breathing · Provide medications as needed for BP, heart rate and rhythm control + IV lidocaine 1.5 mg/kg + 1 mg/min |

↓

- Epinephrine 1 mg IV, repeat every 3 to 5 min (follow with 50 ml NS flush)
- Consider high dose epinephrine (0.1 mg/kg) IV every 3 to 5 minutes
- Consider sodium bicarbonate 1 mEq/kg IV if hyperkalemia known or suspected

↓

- Defibrillate at 360 joules up to 3 times in a row
- Administer lidocaine 1-1.5 mg/kg IV. Repeat in 3-5 min to maximum of 3 mg/kg

↓

- Defibrillate at 360 joules, 30-60 seconds after each dose of medication

↓

- Consider bretylium 5 mg/kg IV, with repeat dose of 10 mg/kg in 5 minutes
- Consider MgSO$_4$ 1-2 g IV if torsades de pointes or suspected hypomagnesemia
- Consider procainamide 30 mg/min to maximum of 17 mg/kg for refractory VF
- Sodium bicarbonate (1-2 mEq/kg IV) is *probably* helpful if known preexisting bicarbonate-responsive acidosis, overdose with tricyclic antidepressants, or to alkalinize the urine in specific drug overdoses
- Sodium bicarbonate (1-2 mEq/kg) is *possibly* helpful if intubated and continued long arrest interval, upon return of spontaneous circulation after a long arrest

Pulseless Electrical Activity (PEA)

- Continue CPR
- Intubate immediately
- Obtain IV access

- If possible, assess cardiac motion with ultrasound, or blood flow via Doppler US, end-tidal CO_2, or arterial line

Consider Possible Causes and (*Treatment*)

- Hypovolemia (*volume infusion*)
- Hypoxia (*ventilation and oxygen*)
- Cardiac tamponade (*pericardiocentesis*)
- Tension pneumothorax (*needle thoracostomy*)
- Massive pulmonary embolism (*consider surgery or thrombolytics*)
- Massive acute MI (*see page 16-19*)

- Drug overdose (*see specific drugs page 90-106*)
- Hypothermia (*see page 37*)
- Hyperkalemia (*see page 26*)
- Acidosis (*sodium bicarbonate 1 mEq/kg IV is probably helpful if known bicarbonate responsive acidosis or tricyclic overdose, or need to alkalinize urine*)

- Administer epinephrine 1 mg IV, repeat q 3-5 minutes
- Administer sodium bicarbonate 1 mEq/kg if known or suspected hyperkalemia
- Consider epinephrine 0.1 mg/kg IV if unresponsive to 1 mg dose

- Administer atropine 1 mg IV if heart rate < 60 beats/min or relative bradycardia
- Repeat atropine 1 mg IV q 3-5 minutes to a total of 0.03-0.04 mg/kg

Asystole

- CPR, obtain IV access, intubate

- Confirm asystole – check 2nd lead

Consider Possible Causes and (Treatment)

- Hypoxia (*intubate, administer O_2*)
- ↓ or ↑ K^+ (*see page 25,26*)
- Acidosis (*sodium bicarbonate 1 mEq/kg for bicarbonate responsive acidosis, overdose with tricyclics or to alkalinize urine in specific drug overdoses*)

- Hypothermia (*see page 37*)
- Drug overdose (*see page 90-106*)

- Consider early transcutaneous pacing simultaneously with drug administration.
- Administer epinephrine 1 mg IV, q 3-5 minutes (consider dose of 0.1 mg/kg).

- Administer atropine 1 mg IV q 3-5 minutes to a total of 0.03-0.04 mg/kg.
- Consider bicarbonate if bicarbonate responsive acidosis, tricyclic overdose, or to alkalinize urine or possibly if prolonged cardiac arrest.
- STOP resuscitation if asystolic > 20-30 min, and no reversible cause found.

Acid Base Disorders

Anion Gap	• $Na^+ - (Cl^- + HCO_3^-)$ *Normal* = 8-16 mEq/L
Osmolal gap	• measured – calculated osmolality *Normal* = 0-10 mOsm/L
Calculated Osmolality	• $2 \times Na^+ + (glucose/18) + (BUN/2.8) + (ethanol/4.6) + (methanol/2.6) + (ethylene glycol/5) + (acetone/5.5) + (isopropanol/5.9)$

Causes of ↑Anion Gap		Causes of ↓Anion Gap	Causes of ↑Osmol Gap

Methanol
Uremia
Diabetes
Paraldehyde
Iron, INH
	Lactate
	Ethanol, ethylene glycol
	Salicylates, starvation
		Lithium,
		Multiple myeloma
		Albumin loss in
		  nephrotic syndrome
			Alcohols (methanol,
			  ethylene glycol,
			  isopropanol)
			Sugars (glycerol,
			  mannitol)
			Ketones (acetone)

MUDPILES

	Primary Disorder	Normal Compensation
Acid Base Rules of Compensation	Metabolic Acidosis	$PCO_2 = (1.5 \times HCO_3^- + 8) \pm 2$
	Acute Respiratory Acidosis	↑$\Delta HCO_3^- = (0.1 \times \Delta PCO_2\uparrow)$
	Chronic Respiratory Acidosis	↑$\Delta HCO_3^- = (0.4 \times \Delta PCO_2\uparrow)$
	Metabolic Alkalosis	$PCO_2 = (0.9 \times HCO_3^- + 9) \pm 2$
	Acute Respiratory Alkalosis	↓$\Delta HCO_3^- = (0.2 \times \Delta PCO_2\downarrow)$
	Chronic Respiratory Alkalosis	↓$\Delta HCO_3^- = (0.4 \times \Delta PCO_2\downarrow)$

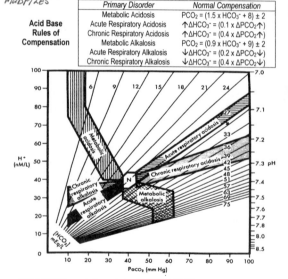

ACID BASE MAP - used with permission *JAMA* 1973; 223: 270.

Anaphylaxis

Anaphylaxis Treatment

Drug	Dose	Route	Indications
epinephrine	0.01	SC/IM	mild to moderate symptoms
	mg/kg[1]	IV	airway compromise, severe hypotension (dilute 3 ml of 1:10,000 of epinephrine in 10 ml NS and administer IV over several minutes, followed by a drip (page 128) for SEVERE reactions only[1])
normal saline	20 ml/kg	IV	hypotension
Solu-Medrol	2 mg/kg	IV	moderate/severe symptoms
Benadryl	1 mg/kg max 50mg	IV/IM	moderate/severe symptoms
cimetidine	5 mg/kg	IV/IM	if no wheezing (bronchoconstricts)
glucagon	1-2 mg	IV	if patient taking a β-blocker
albuterol	0.2-0.4 mg	nebulized	bronchospasm
racemic epi.	0.25-.5 ml	nebulized	stridor

[1] Use extreme caution with IV route as severe life-threatening complications can occur.

Bee Sting : Remove stinger, rinse, apply ice. Consider small dose of epinephrine 0.005 ml/kg locally if not an end-organ site (fingers, toes, nose, etc.).

Unresponsive anaphylaxis consider:
  (1) Hereditary angioedema (consider fresh frozen plasma, or *Danazol*),
  (2) β-blocker use (consider glucagon 1-2 mg IV or SC)
  (3) An alternate cause for symptoms (e.g. bleeding, sepsis)

Anesthesia & Airway Management

Anatomic Indicators of Difficult Airway

- ≤ 40 mm from chin to hyoid cartilage (≤ three finger-breadths)
- ≤ 40 mm from upper to lower incisors (≤ three finger-breadths)
- large tongue or inability to see uvula and tonsillar pillars with mouth opened
- limited hinge movement of temporomandibular joint (e.g. rheumatoid arthritis, inflammatory trismus from deep space infection, or mandibular fracture)
- congenital cleft, maxillary or mandibular anomalies
- protruding maxillary incisors or maxillofacial trauma
- upper airway obstruction or bleeding (trauma, infection, burn, inhalation injury)

Prediction of Difficulty of Endotracheal Intubation *Can Anaesth Soc J* 1985; 32: 429.	Class	Anatomy of airway (Mallampati)	Difficulty[1]
	I	Visible soft palate, tonsillar pillars	Minimal
	II	Visible soft palate, tonsillar pillars	Moderate
	III	Visible soft palate only	Severe
	IV	Visible hard palate only	Severe

[1] on laryngoscopy, glottis is visible in > 99% class I, 90% class II, and < 70% class III&IV airways

Rapid Sequence Intubation Steps And Drugs

Prepare Equipment

- ready 2 wall suction devices with Yankauer tips, check laryngoscope light
- appropriate ET tube (7-7.5 mm for adult females and 7.5-8 mm internal diameter for males) and back-up 1 size smaller with stylet, check ET cuff

Patient Preparation after Airway Assessment above

- raise bed to comfortable height (e.g., patient's nose at intubator's xiphoid)
- prepare alternate airway plan: jet ventilator, tracheostomy, cricothyrotomy
- ensure pulse oximeter and cardiac monitor attached and working
- specify personnel for (1) cricoid pressure, (2) neck immobilization if trauma, (3) handling ET tube, (4) watching O_2 sat & cardiac monitors, and (5) medications
- position head appropriately (sniffing position if no trauma)
- draw up all drugs in syringes and ensure secure IV access is available
- preoxygenate with 100% oxygen for at least 3-4 minutes (if possible)
- perform Sellick maneuver (cricoid pressure)

Medication

- lidocaine 1.5 mg/kg IV if head injured to blunt the intracranial pressure response to laryngoscopy
- consider use of defasciculating agent IV if succinylcholine will be administered (then wait 1.5 to 2 minutes)
- administer sedating, then paralyzing agent IV (see page 9)

Drugs for Rapid Sequence Intubation

Agent	Dose IV	Onset	Key Properties
Defasciculating drug	*(mg/kg)*	*(min)*	
rocuronium[1]	0.06	2-3	
succinylcholine	0.1	3	↑ICP, GI, and eye pressures
vecuronium	0.01	3	minimal tachycardia
Sedating drug	*(mg/kg)*	*(min)*	
etomidate[2]	0.3-0.4	1-2	minimal blood pressure decrease
fentanyl	2-10 µg/kg	1-2	↑ICP, chest wall rigidity
ketamine	1-2	< 1	↑BP, ICP, GI, eye pressures
midazolam	0.1-0.2	1-3	causes hypotension
propofol	1-2.5	< 1	hypotension
thiopental	2-5	< 1	hypotension, bronchospasm
Paralyzing drug	*(mg/kg)*	*(min)*	
succinylcholine[3]	1-2	< 1	↑ICP, GI, and eye pressures
rocuronium	0.6-1.2	< 1	tachycardia, mild histamine release
vecuronium	0.1 - 0.3	1-4	prolonged action

1→2→3 Standard drug sequence if no contraindications exist

Steps to Perform After Intubation	1. Check tube placement (breath sounds, CO_2 detector) 2. Inflate cuff, then release cricoid pressure 3. Normal depth of any ET tube (cm) is approximately is 3 X ET tube internal diameter (mm) from midtrachea to incisors 4. Reassess patient's BP, pulse, pulse oximetry 5. Obtain CXR to verify correct ET depth (between T2-T4) 6. Consider long acting sedative and paralytics

Guidelines for Initiating Mechanical Ventilation in Adults

Item	Initial Setting	Comments
Mode	Assist control	Ventilator assists if patient breathes on own
	Controlled,	Patient cannot breathe on own
		(e.g., completely sedated or paralyzed)
	IMV, SIMV	Set rate that allows patient to breathe on own
Tidal Volume	10-15 ml/kg	5-7 ml/kg if ↑peak airway pressures (e.g. asthma)
Rate	12-14/minute	
FiO_2	50-100%	Reduce as soon as possible to < 50%
PEEP	None	Start at 5 cm H_2O if paO_2 < 60 & $FiO_2 \geq$ 50%
I:E	1:2	Reverse ratio of $\geq$ 2:1 for ARDS, pulmonary edema
Insp. flow	50L/min	If too slow, causes inadequate exhalation
Insp. pause	None	Leads to even ventilation, and air trapping
Peak pressure	50 cm H_2O	Start at 20-30 cm if pressure cycled ventilator
Exp. retard	None	May prevent premature collapse of airway

Burns and Burn Therapy

**Estimation of
Total Body Surface Area Burned**

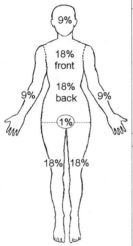

**Admission and Transfer Criteria for
Patients with Significant Burns**

Admission Criteria[1]
Burn TBSA ≥ 15% (2nd + 3rd degree)
Burn TBSA ≥ 10% (age > 50 years)
Burn TBSA ≥ 2-5% (3rd degree)
Burns to hands, feet, face, perineum
Minor chemical burn
Associated carbon monoxide poisoning
Inadequate family support or known or suspected abuse
Severe underlying medical disease (e.g. emphysema, coronary artery disease, diabetes, renal insufficiency)

Transfer to Burn Center[1]
Burn TBSA ≥ 25% (2nd + 3rd degree)
Burn TBSA ≥ 20% (age > 50 years)
Burn TBSA ≥ 10% (3rd degree)
3rd degree hands, feet, face, perineum
Major chemical or electrical burn
Respiratory tract injury
Associated major trauma
Circumferential limb burns

[1]TBSA - total body surface area

Fluid Resuscitation in Burn Victims

Parkland formula	• Lactated ringers 4 ml/kg/%burn BSA[1] in 1st 24 hours + maintenance fluid, with ½ over 1st 8 h, & ½ over next 16 h
Alternatives	• *Amended Parkland formula*: for ED stays < 8 hours. IV rate over maintenance (ml/h) = [weight(kg) X burn BSA%] ÷ 4 • *Carvajal's formula*: Carvajal's solution 5,000 ml/m² of burn + maintenance 2000 ml/m² in 1st 24h , with ½ over the 1st 8 hours and ½ over the subsequent 16 hours.

[1]BSA = body surface area

ECG Diagnosis of Arrhythmia, Blocks, and Medical Disorders

Normal Adult ECG (small box: 1 mm = 0.04 sec; large box: 5 mm = 0.20 sec)
- *P wave* - < 0.10 sec, ↑ in I, II, and ↓ in aVR.; *PR interval* - 0.12 - 0.20 sec.
- *QRS complex* - 0.05-0.10 seconds; normally ↑ in II, V5, V6; ↓ in aVR,V1; transition zone in V3; ↑ or ↓ in aVL, aVF,III; left chest leads height is < 27 mm.
- *Q wave*- normally < 0.04 seconds, and < 25% height of following R.
- *QT interval* - 0.34-0.42 seconds or 40% of RR interval
- *QTc* (corrected QT) = QT interval/square root of R-R. Normal < 0.47 seconds.
- *T wave* - ↑ in I, V6, and ↓ in aVR; Normal ↓ T waves may be found in III, aVF, aVL,V1 : Abnormal ↓ T waves may signify LVH (esp V6), LBBB, ischemia, MI.
- *Axis* : Normal: -30 degrees to +100 degrees. *Left axis deviation* (LAD): -30 to -90 degrees. *Right axis deviation* (RAD): +100 to +180 or -90 to -180 degrees.

Conduction Blocks
- *1st degree AV block* - PR interval > 0.2 seconds, P precedes each QRS.
- *2nd degree AV block* - (type 1/Wenckebach) - increasing PR interval until QRS dropped. (type 2) - QRS dropped without increasing PR interval.
- *3rd degree AV block* - P and QRS are independent. Fixed P-P intervals.
- *Right bundle branch block* (RBBB) (1) QRS ≥ 0.12 sec (± 0.1-0.12 sec) (2) R-R'/R-S-R' in V1/V2 (3) ST-T opposite to terminal QRS (4) S in I, aVL,V5,V6.
- *Left bundle branch block* (LBBB) - (1) QRS ≥ 0.12 sec (2) R or R-R' in I, aVL, or V6; (3) negative wave (rS or QS) in V1, (4) no septal Q wave of 0.01 or 0.02 in I and V6. (5) ST-T waves directed opposite to the terminal 0.04 sec QRS.
- *Anterior Hemiblock* - LAD < - 45, QRS 0.10-0.12 sec, small Q in I, aVL; R in II, III, and aVF; terminal R in aVR.
- *Posterior Hemiblock* - RAD; QRS 0.10-0.12 sec; S in I; Q in II, III, aVF.

Hypertrophy
- *Right Atrial* - P > 2.5 mm in II or large diaphasic P in V1 (tall initial phase)
- *Left Atrial* - diphasic P in V1 with large terminal downward phase.
- *Right Ventricular* (RVH) - RAD > 100, incomplete RBBB in V1; R>S - V1; R > 5 mm - V1; decreasing R in V1 to V4; ST depression + flipped T's V1-V3, ± RAH.
- *Left Ventricular* (LVH) – Romhilt and Estes criteria

Romhilt and Estes criteria for Diagnosing LVH	Points
QRS with largest R or S in limb leads ≥ 20 mm **or** S in V1 or V2 ≥ 30 mm **or** R in V5 or V6 ≥ 30 mm	3
ST-T downsloping without digitalis (3 points) or with digitalis (1 point)	1 or 3
Left atrial enlargement	3
Left axis deviation < 30 degrees or more	2
QRS duration > 0.9 seconds	1
Intrinsicoid deflection (time from onset QRS to apex R) in V5 and V6 ≥ 0.05 seconds	1
If total points ≥ 5 = definite LVH, total points = 4 signifies probable LVH	

Myocardial injury and ischemia.

Location	Leads	Coronary Arteries involved
Anterior	V2-V4	Left anterior descending (LAD)
Anteroseptal	V1-V4	LAD
Anterolateral	V1-V6, I, aVL	LAD, diagonal
Inferior	II, III, aVF	Right coronary, circumflex
Lateral	I, aVL, V5, V6	Circumflex, diagonal
Posterior	large R -V1,V2,V3, reciprocal ST ↓	Right coronary artery

ST ↑ ≥ 1 mm = injury/infarcton,Q > 0.04 sec = infarction, T flattening/inversion = ischemia.

Typical ECG Findings in Acute MI

- Early on, a marked increase in R wave voltage may occur.
- Prominent (hyperacute) T waves with normal direction occur early (esp. > 5 mm). T waves are peaked and symmetric ~ church steeple (± wider than ↑K).
- ST segment elevation that is either convex > concave upward.
- Q waves > 0.04 sec other than leads aVR + V1 and T wave flattening/inversion.

Predictive Value of Initial EKG in Acute MI	Sensitivity	Specificity
• New Q waves or ST segment elevation	40%	> 90%
• Above or ST segment depression	75%	80%
• Any of above or prior ischemia/infarction changes	85%	76%
• Any of above or nonspecific ST-T changes	90%	65%

Ann Emerg Med 1990; 19: 1359

Diagnosis of Acute MI in Presence of Left Bundle Branch Block

Criteria for Diagnosis of Acute MI	Points
• ST segment elevation ≥ 1 mm concordant (same direction) as QRS	5
• ST segment depression ≥ 1 mm in leads V1, V2, or V3	3
• ST segment elevation ≥ 5 mm and discordant (opposite) with QRS	2

Total ≥ 3 is 36-78% sensitive, 90-96% specific for acute MI. *New Engl J Med* 1996;334: 481.

ECG Findings in Pericarditis

- ST segment elevation is typically diffuse involving elevation in I, II, and III or at least 2 bipolar limb leads and precordial leads V1 through V6 or V2 through V6.
- ST depression is common in aVR, and may occur in II and V1. ST segment ↑ is typically concave upward and ≤ 5 mm in height. Pathologic Q waves are rare.
- Up to 82% exhibit PR segment depression.
- Sequence of ST-T changes: (1) initial ST ↑, (2) ST returns to baseline before T waves flip (↓) (3) T wave ↓ is usually ≤ 5 mm and (4) T waves normalize.
- Low voltage QRS or electrical alternans suggests pericardial fluid.
- ± Height of ST segment/T wave > 0.25 in V5, V6, or I.

ECG Findings in Benign Early Repolarization

- Typically, concave upward appearance to ST segments.
- ST segment elevations are almost always ≤ 5 mm and typically ≤ 2 mm.
- ST segment elevations are more often found in V3-V6 than in V1 and V2.
- Occasionally can be associated with reciprocal ST segment depressions.
- Prominent T waves ≥ 7 mm may be found.
- Notched J point (junction of QRS and ST segment) is typical.
- Pathologic Q waves are rare.

ECG Findings in Medical Disorders

Disorder	ECG Finding
COPD	RAD (negative lead I), overall low voltage, RAH ± RBBB
Pulmonary emboli	ST/T wave changes, RAD, RBBB. large S in I or Q in III
Hyperkalemia	Peaked T's, wide then flat P's, wide QRS and QT, sine wave
Hypokalemia	Flat T waves, U waves, U > T waves, ST depression
Calcium	High calcium - short QT, low calcium - long QT interval
Pericarditis	Flat/concave ST ↑, PR ↓, ↓ voltage
Digoxin effect	Downward curve of ST segment, flat/inverted T's, shorter QT
Digoxin toxicity	PVC's (60%), AV block (20%), Ectopic SVT (25%), V tach.
Hypothyroidism	Sinus bradycardia, low voltage, ST ↓, flat or inverted T waves
Hyperthyroidism	Sinus tachycardia

Arrhythmias

- Multifocal atrial tachycardia - 3 or more different P waves, normal QRS complex and associated with COPD, hypoxia, digoxin or theophylline toxicity, or ASCVD.
- Paroxysmal atrial tachycardia - P's occur before each QRS with rate 150-250.
- Paroxysmal supraventricular tachycardia - Rate 120-250, either narrow or wide QRS (if Bundle Branch Block or pre-excitation), P waves may be visible or hidden in QRS complex.
- Atrial flutter - atrial rate 200-400 saw tooth pattern (esp. leads II and III), common ventricular rate of 150 due to 2:1 block (with atrial rate of 300).
- Atrial fibrillation - highly irregular rhythm, no discernible P waves, ventricular rate may be rapid or slow depending on conduction.
- Ventricular tachycardia - ≥ 3 premature ventricular beats in a row, broad QRS rhythm at rate of 100-250/min. May be associated with fusion beats, AV dissociation, LAD, precordial concordance.
- Ventricular fibrillation (VF) - irregular chaotic baseline, no beats, no BP.
- Torsades de pointes - twisting QRS, prolonged QT interval, may progress to VF.

Treatment of Paroxysmal Supraventricular Tachycardia in Adults

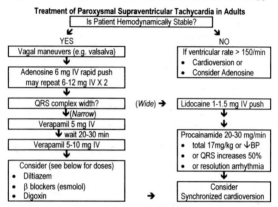

| | Is Patient Hemodynamically Stable? | |

YES

- Vagal maneuvers (e.g. valsalva)
- Adenosine 6 mg IV rapid push may repeat 6-12 mg IV X 2
- QRS complex width? →(*Narrow*)
- Verapamil 5 mg IV ↓ wait 20-30 min
- Verapamil 5-10 mg IV
- Consider (see below for doses)
  - Diltiazem
  - β blockers (esmolol)
  - Digoxin

(Wide) →

NO

If ventricular rate > 150/min
- Cardioversion or
- Consider Adenosine

Lidocaine 1-1.5 mg IV push

Procainamide 20-30 mg/min
- total 17mg/kg or ↓BP
- or QRS increases 50%
- or resolution arrhythmia

→ Consider Synchronized cardioversion

Supraventricular Tachycardia (SVT), Atrial Fibrillation (AFib) and Atrial Flutter (AFlut) Treatment Options (if clinically stable)[1]

- adenosine (*Adenocard*) 6 mg IV. May repeat 12 mg IV q 2 min X 2 doses. Do not use if 2nd or 3rd degree AV block, sick sinus syndrome, or on dipyridamole. Worsens bronchospasm if asthma, COPD, or theophylline use. (SVT)
- digoxin (*Lanoxin*) 0.5 mg IV or PO at 0 + 4 h, + 0.25 mg PO at 8 + 12 h.(AFib/AFlut)
- diltiazem (*Cardizem*) 20 mg (0.25 mg/kg) IV over 2 min. Repeat 30 mg (0.35 mg/kg) IV 15 min after 1st dose prn. Drip at 5-15 mg/h prn. (SVT, AFib/AFlut)
- esmolol (*Brevibloc*)
  (1) Load 500µg/kg IV over 1 min followed by infusion of 50µg/kg/min X 4 min.
  (2) If no response, 500µg/kg IV over 1 min, then 100µg/kg/min X 4 minutes.
  (3) If needed, repeat 500µg/kg over 1 min while increasing infusion by 50µg/kg/min until maximum of 200µg/kg/min. Esmolol half life is 9 min.
  (4) Once OK response, do not change rate > 25µg/kg/min and do not rebolus.
- magnesium 1-2 gm IV over 15 min. (SVT, AFib/AFlut)
- metoprolol (*Lopressor*) 1mg/min IV (max 7.5 mg). (SVT, AFib/AFlut)
- propanolol (*Inderal*) 1-3 mg IV at 1 mg/min. (SVT, AFib/AFlut)
- verapamil[2] (*Calan*) 5-10 mg IV over 2 minutes. May repeat 10 mg IV over 2 minutes, 30 minutes after 1st dose. Avoid if wide complex. (SVT, AFib/AFlut)

[1] Treatment recommendations are only for narrow complex tachyarrhythmias, in clinically stable patients. If patient is hypotension, or in extremis cardiovert immediately.

[2] Do not use at same time as IV β-blockers.

Differentiation of Wide complex SVT from Ventricular Tachycardia

Feature	Suggests SVT	Suggests VT[1]
Age	< 35 years	> 50 years
Prior MI		95% specific for VT
Past Hx	Prior SVT	Angina, Congestive heart failure
Symptoms and BP	Not useful differentiator	Not useful differentiator
AV dissociation		specific for VT
QRS duration		≥ 0.14 seconds (≥ 0.16 if LBBB)
QRS axis		-90 to ± 180 degrees (NW axis) or concordance in all precordial leads
V1 or V2 if LBBB		R > .03 sec, or > .07 sec to S nadir
V6 if LBBB		QR or QS
V1 if RBBB	triphasic QRS or R'>R	Monophasic R, QR, RS
V6 if RBBB	triphasic QRS	R/S < 1, QS, QR

[1] Absence of features suggesting VT DOES NOT imply that SVT is more likely. No single feature is 100% accurate at differentiating between these two disorders.

Emerg Med Clin N Am 1995; 13: 903.

Algorithm for Diagnosis of Wide Complex QRS Tachycardia

Is RS complex absent in all precordial leads?	Yes→	Ventricular tachycardia
No ↓		
Is R to S interval > 100 ms in 1 precordial lead?	Yes→	Ventricular tachycardia
No ↓		
Is Atrio-ventricular dissociation present?	Yes→	Ventricular tachycardia
No ↓		
Morphology criteria for VT present both in precordial leads V1-V2 and V6 (see above)	Yes→	Ventricular tachycardia
No ↓		
SVT with aberrant conduction is likely		

The sensitivity and specificity of algorithm was 99 and 97%, respectively in a single study. Accuracy is lower in those taking anti-dysrhythmics. *Circulation* 1991; 83: 1649.

Management of Ventricular Tachycardia

- If no pulse, immediately defibrillate & treat as ventricular fibrillation (page 4)
- If hypotension, pulmonary edema, depressed consciousness or chest pain, immediately cardiovert (synchronized) with 50j, doubling to maximum 360j.
- If hemodynamically stable, (1) lidocaine 1 mg/kg IV, then 0.5 mg/min q 5-10 min up to 3 mg/kg or rhythm stops. (2) if persistent VT, procainamide 20-30 mg/min IV to maximum 17 mg/kg or hypotension, or QRS widens 50%, or rhythm stops, then bretylium if rhythm persists (3) once terminated, lidocaine infusion 1-4 mg/min IV or procainide 1-4 mg/min, if procainimide terminated rhythm.

CARDIAC PARAMETERS AND FORMULAS	Normal Values
Cardiac output (CO) = heart rate x stroke volume	4-8 L/min
Cardiac index (CI) = CO/BSA	2.8-4.2 L/min/m^2
Mean arterial pressure (MAP) = (Systolic BP-Diastolic BP)/3 +Diastolic BP	80-100 mmHg
Systemic vascular resistance (SVR) = (MAP-CVP)x(80)/CO	800-1200 dynes/sec/cm^2
Pulmonary vascular resistance (PVR) = (PAM-PCWP)(80)/CO	45-120 dynes/sec/cm^2
Central venous pressure (CVP)	5-12 cm H20
Pulmonary artery systolic pressure	20-30 mmHg
Pulmonary artery diastolic pressure	10-15 mmHg
Pulmonary artery mean pressure	15-20 mmHg
Pulmonary capillary wedge pressure (PCWP)	8-12 mmHg

Assessment and Management of Acute Pulmonary Edema

Most Common Acute Pulmonary Edema Precipitants

•	Worsening CHF	26%	• Dysrhythmia	9%
•	Ischemia without infarction	21%	• Medication noncompliance	7%
•	Subendocardial infarction	16%	• Dietary indiscretion	3%
•	Transmural infarction	10%	• Valvular insufficiency	3%

Treatment Options

- Oxygen 100% - consider continuous positive airway pressure (CPAP) or intubation.
- Nitroglycerin If BP normal or ↑, start IV rate at 10-20 µg/min and titrate to (1) symptom relief (2) fall in MAP of 30% or (3) systolic BP (SBP) falls to 90 mmHg.
- Furosemide (Lasix) 40-80 mg IV to venodilate and reduce preload by diuresis.
- Morphine sulfate - 2-8 mg IV, titrate to decrease catecholamine effect/afterload.
- Sodium nitroprusside (Nipride) 0.5-10µg/kg/min IV if extremely elevated BP. 2nd line agent if ischemia is not prominent and continuous invasive monitoring.
- Consider captopril 12.5 mg PO or enalapril 1.25 mg IV for hypertension.
- Dobutamine 2-20µg/kg/min may be added to increase contractility if normal SBP.
- If SBP < 90 mmHg and signs of shock consider
  1. Normal saline 250-500 ml IV , especially useful if right ventricular infarction.
  2. dopamine 2.5 - 20µg/kg/min IV:
  - at 1-2 µg/kg/min renal and mesenteric blood flow are increased.
  - at 2-10 µg/kg/min myocardial contractility increases via β1 stimulation.
  - at > 10 µg/kg/min α-adrenergic stimulation & vasoconstriction occur.
  3. dobutamine 2-20µg/kg/min IV may be used if no shock, but SBP 70-100 mm Hg
  4. norepinephrine 0.5-30 µg/min IV if dopamine at > 20µg/kg/min is needed to maintain pressure > 70-80 mm Hg. Infuse through central line.
  5. amrinone 0.75 mg/kg then 5-15 µg/kg/min if other drugs fail.
- If refractory pulmonary edema, exclude volume loss, valvular insufficiency (echocardiography), and arrhythmia.

Diagnosis of Acute Myocardial Infarction (MI)

Of patients presenting to the ED with acute chest pain, ~ 15% will harbor acute ischemic heart disease. The table below details the predictive values for diagnosis of Acute Myocardial Infarction and does NOT detail the risk for Unstable Angina.

Utility of Various Tests for Diagnosis of Acute MI

Diagnostic Test	Sensitivity	Specificity	PPV[k]	NPV[k]
12 lead ECG (liberal criteria)[a]	94-99	19-27	21	98
12 lead ECG (intermediate criteria)[b]	69-75	83-86	44	95
12 lead ECG (strict criteria)[c]	38-44	97-98	76	91
15 lead ECG (+V8,V9,V4R)	55-60[i]	97-98		
22 lead ECG (many AP thorax leads)	88[i]	---		
ECG stress test[d]	68[j]	77		
CK-MB enzymes over 24 h	100	98		
1st CK-MB, pain onset < 4 h prior	41	88		
1st CK-MB, pain onset > 4 h prior	63	90		
Serial CK-MB isoform, pain = 4 h[e]	56	93	Data sources:
Serial CK-MB isoform, pain = 6 h[e]	96	94	NHAAP report
CK-MB at 0,1,2,3 h after ED arrival[f]	80	94	*Ann Emerg Med*
Myoglobin, pain onset = 2 h	89	96	1997; 29(1)
Myoglobin, pain onset 12-24 h	59	95	and
Troponin T, pain onset = 2 h	33	100	*Acad Emerg*
Troponin T, pain onset = 6 h	78	99	*Med* 1997;4:13
Troponin T, pain onset 12-24 h	93	99	and
Echocardiography[g]	86-88	78-82	*Ann Emerg Med*
Sestamibi (technetium 99m scan)[h]	94-100	83-92	1992; 21: 504

[a] nonspecific ST segment or T wave changes abnormal but not diagnostic of ischemia; Or ischemia, strain, or infarction known or not known to be old.

[b] ST segment elevation/depression, or T wave abnormalities consistent with ischemia or strain, not known to be old.

[c] ST segment elevation or pathologic Q waves not known to be old.

[d] Predictive values for presence of significant coronary artery disease, not AMI.

[e] CK-MB isoforms were collected every 30-60 minutes for at least 6 hours after symptom onset when studied. Criteria for AMI diagnosis: MB2 > 1U/L or MB2/MB1 > 1.5.

[f] Sensitivity/specificity if > 6 hours from pain onset. Numbers are lower if < 6 hours.

[g] Sensitivity/specificity if obtained during chest pain.

[h] Must have ongoing chest pain and no nitrate or β blocker administered before test.

[i] Sensitivity using criteria strict ECG above

[j] Sensitivity is higher for three vessel disease and lower if LVH noted on ECG.

[k] NPV - negative predictive value, PPV - positive predictive value

**American College of Cardiology/American Heart Association (ACC/AHA)
Recommendations for Thrombolytic Therapy in Acute MI**

Class	Recommendation
I	• ST elevation > 0.1 mV in ≥ 2 contiguous leads **AND** time to therapy of ≤ 12 hours **AND** age < 75 years • New bundle branch block **AND** history highly suggestive of acute MI
II a	• ST elevation > 0.1 mV in ≥ 2 contiguous leads **AND** age ≥ 75 years
II b	• ST elevation > 0.1 mV in ≥ 2 contiguous leads + time to therapy 12-24 h • Presenting systolic BP > 180 mm Hg or diastolic BP > 110 mm Hg with **high-risk MI**. An attempt to lower BP 1st with β blockers, or nitrates is recommended but not proven to lower risk of intracranial hemorrhage. **High risk MI** - female, age > 70 years, prior MI, atrial fibrillation, anterior MI, rales in > 1/3 of lung fields, low BP sinus tachycardia or diabetes.
III	• ST elevation > 0.1mV in ≥ 2 contiguous leads + time to therapy > 24 h • ST segment depression only

Class I - evidence or general agreement that treatment is beneficial, useful, & effective.
Class II - conflicting evidence or a divergence of opinion about usefulness or efficacy.
    (IIa) - weight of evidence is in favor of efficacy. (IIb) - efficacy is less well established.
Class III - evidence or agreement that treatment is not useful and may be harmful.
J Am Coll Cardiol 1996; 28: 1328.

Absolute Contraindications to Thrombolytic Use

Prior hemorrhagic stroke at any time	Active internal bleeding (not menses)
Stroke/TIA in past 1 year, CNS neoplasm	Suspect aortic dissection, pericarditis

Relative Contraindications or Cautions to Thrombolytic Use

BP > 180/110 on presentation	Noncompressible vascular puncture
Current anticoagulation (INR ≥ 2-3) or known bleeding diathesis	Internal bleeding in past 2-4 weeks
	Streptokinase use (1-2 years), tPA is OK
History or prior stroke or known CNS pathology not included above	Recent trauma (<2-4 weeks) (head/spine trauma, CPR > 10 min, major surgery)
Pregnancy, active peptic ulcer	History of chronic severe hypertension

J Am Coll Cardiol 1996; 28: 1328.

Thrombolytic Dose and Choice of Agent

Agent[1]	Dose	Criteria
r-PA	• 10 U IV over 2 min, repeat dose in 30 min • Administer heparin as detailed for tPA	• See tPA below
t-PA	• 15 mg bolus + 0.75 mg/kg (max 50 mg) over 30 min + 0.50 mg/kg (max. 35 mg) over 60 min + heparin 5000 U bolus + 1000U/h. PTT goal = 65-80 sec.	• Age ≤ 75 years • Anterior Wall or _possibly_ large inferior-lateral MI • Symptoms ≤ 4 hours
SK	• 1.5 million U. IV over 1 hour	• All others (unless prior SK)

r-PA – reteplase (Retavase); t-PA – tissue plasminogen activator or alteplase (Activase); SK – streptokinase (Streptase)   GUSTO. New Engl J Med 1993; 329: 637.

ACC/AHA Guidelines for Adjunctive Drug Therapy in Acute MI

Agent	Class	Recommendation
ACE inhibitors	I	• Within 1st 24 h of MI with ST elevation in ≥ 2 anterior precordial leads or CHF without ↓BP, or contraindication
	II a	• All other patients within 24 hours of suspected MI
	II b	• Recovered from MI + normal/mildly abnormal LV[1] function
Aspirin	I	• Begin immediately and continue indefinitely
	II b	• If allergy, substitute dipyridamole or ticlopidine
β-blockers	I	• Within 12 hours of MI or with ongoing, recurrent pain
	II b	• Non Q wave MI
	III	• Heart failure, bradycardia, or other contraindication
Ca^{+2} channel blockers	I	• No class I indications
Heparin (low molecular weight ± superior)	I	• Patients undergoing PTCA[2] or surgery
	II a	• Use IV for 48 hours if alteplase use
	II b	• Subcutaneous use if nonselective thrombolytics administered, and low risk for emboli until ambulatory
Lidocaine	I	• Sustained monomorphic ventricular tachycardia (VT) not associated with angina, hypotension, or CHF
	II a	• For 6-24 hours after ventricular fibrillation/tachycardia
	III	• Prophylaxis with thrombolytics, isolated PVC's, couplets, accelerated idioventricular rhythm, nonsustained VT
Magnesium	I	• No class I recommendations
	II a	• Treating low K$^+$ or low Mg^{+2}, or torsades de pointes
Nitroglycerin	I	• 1st 24-48 h in acute MI with CHF, large anterior infarct, persistent ischemia, or hypertension
	II b	• 1st 24-48 h after MI without↓BP, brady or tachycardia
	III	• Systolic BP < 90 mmHg, or heart rate < 50 beats/minute

[1]LV-left ventricle, [2]PTCA – percutaneous coronary angioplasty.

J Am Coll Cardiol 1996; 28: 1328.

Adjunctive Therapy in Acute MI

Agent	Dose	Contraindication
Aspirin	160-325 mg PO	Allergy, severe bleeding diathesis
Atenolol (Tenormin)	5 mg IV q 5 min X 2, then 100 mg PO q day	Bradycardia, ↓BP, CHF, 2nd or 3rd degree AV block, asthma , COPD
Heparin	80 U/kg IV, then 18U/kg/h	Allergy, bleeding diathesis
Magnesium	1-4 g IV over 15-20 min	Renal failure
Metoprolol (Lopressor)	5 mg IV q 5 min X 3, then 50 mg PO q 6 hours	Bradycardia, ↓BP, CHF, 2nd or 3rd degree AV block, asthma , COPD

Abdominal Aortic Aneurysm (AAA)

AAA-diameter ≥1.5X adjacent aorta or ≥ 3cm

Risk factors: male, family history (25% risk if AAA in sibling/parent), ↑ age, smoking, ↑BP peripheral or collagen vascular disease.

Radiologic evaluation: Plain films show calcified aortic wall in ~ 60%. Angiography can miss AAA with mural thrombus. US detects all AAA's but only leakage in 4%. CT identifies 100% of AAA's & rupture but not aortoenteric & aortovenous fistula, inflammatory aneurysms, & infections. Use MRI instead.

Clinical Features of Ruptured AAA	
Abdominal Pain	77%
Flank or back pain	60%
Vomiting	25%
Syncope	18%
Hematemesis	5%
Known AAA	5%
Pulsatile mass	70%
Abdomen tenderness	41%
Pain, mass, and low BP	30-40%
Absent low ext. pulses	6%
Anuria or abd. bruit	< 1%

Management: (1) If rupture and unstable, resuscitate as needed, go to O.R. for repair (± bedside US) Do not delay repair. (2) If rupture and hemodynamically stable, cardiac monitor, O_2, large bore IV X 2 with NS. Obtain ECG, CXR, CBC, renal function, electrolytes and type and cross for 4-6 units of blood. Immediately notify surgeon. CT or MRI. _Emerg Med Reports 1994; 15: 125._

Thoracic Aortic Dissection

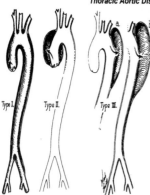

Type I.   Type II.   Type III.

With permission. _J Thorac Cardiovasc Surg_ 1965;49:130.

DeBakey classification	
Type I (ascending + descending), Type II (ascending aorta only), Type III (distal to subclavian artery) [IIIa above & IIIb below diaphragm]	

Stanford classification	
A = DeBakey I & II, B = type III	

Clinical Features	
Chest or back pain	88%
Aortic regurgitation ±CHF	50%
Transitory pulse deficits	50%
Neurologic deficit	20%
Hypotension	20%
Syncope	5%
No pain	12%
Other features include tamponade, acute abdominal pain, hematuria, oliguria, dyspnea, Horner's syndrome, superior vena cava syndrome, GI bleed, hemoptysis.	

J Emerg Med 1997; 15: 859.

Thoracic Aortic Dissection - Diagnosis

CXR Findings		Diagnostic Study	Sensitivity	Specificity
Any abnormality	85%	Transthoracic	-	-
Wide mediastinum	75%	echocardiography	75%	85-90%
Aortic knob abnormalities (Ca^{+2}	-	Angiography	85%	90-95%
separated > 5mm from knob a	-	Conventional CT	65-85%	95-100%
bulge or obliterated knob)	66%	Helical CT	90-100%	95-100%
Irregular aortic contour	38%	Transesophageal		
Displaced trachea or NG tube	-	echocardiography	95-100%	90-97%
Left pleural effusion	27%	MRI	95-100%	95-100

Lancet 1997; 349: 1461; *J Emerg Med* 1997; 15: 859

Management: If unstable, resuscitate & prepare for surgery. If stable, consult surgeon, control pain, BP & HR. Goal = HR of 60-80 & systolic BP = 90-110 mm Hg.

- Labetolol (*Normodyne*) - 0.25 mg/kg IV, double q 15 min up to 2 mg/kg or 300 mg
- Alternately, use a β blocker + Nitroprusside. β blocker choices include (1, 2)
  1. propanolol (*Inderal*) 1 mg IV q 5 min (max dose 0.15 mg/kg) **or**
  2. esmolol (*Breviblock*) - bolus 500 µg/kg and start drip at 50-200 µg/kg/min
  3. sodium nitroprusside (*Nipride*) - 0.5 -10 µg/kg/min.
- Surgery is indicated for most ascending (Stanford A) dissections, but not B.

Syncope

Syncope is a sudden temporary loss of consciousness with a loss of tone and spontaneous recovery. Relatively benign causes include vasodepressor syncope from excess vagal tone, micturation & defecation syncope, orthostatic syncope from dehydration or blood loss and drug induced syncope. Life threatening causes include dysrhythmias, aortic stenosis, MI, pulmonary embolus, vertebrobasilar transient ischemic attacks & cardiac conduction defects.

Cause of syncope in 433 patients			
Cardiac (25%)		**Noncardiac(34%)**	
Vent tachycardia	11%	Orthostasis	10%
Sick sinus	3%	Vasodepressor	8%
Complete heart		Situational	8%
or Mobitz II block	2%	Drugs	2%
SVT	2%	TIA	2%
Aortic stenosis	2%	Seizure	2%
MI, ↓HR	-	Others - each	1%
Carotid sinus	-	UNKNOWN	41%
Aortic dissection	1%	Kapoor. *Medicine*	
Pulmonary	1%	1990; 69: 160.	
embolus			

Diagnosis

Evaluation includes complete examination with rectal to look for occult blood, orthostatic vitals signs, a βhCG in women of child-bearing age, an EKG and pulse oximetry. Further evaluation is guided by the history and physical.

Studies Revealing Syncope Etiology	
History and physical exam	49%
Electrocardiographic monitoring	27%
Electrocardiogram	11%
Cardiac catheterization	7%
Electrophysiologic study	3%
Cerebral angiography	2%
Electroencephalography	1%

Syncope continued...

Management: If a cardiac or any life-threatening cause for syncope is considered, it must either be ruled out definitively in the emergency department or the patient must be admitted to the hospital (on continuous telemetry).

The risk factors listed to the right should increase threshold for admission to the hospital. If 3 out of 4 listed risk factors are present, mortality risk within one year is 58-80%. If no risk factors are present, mortality risk within one year is 4-7%.

Martin. *Ann Emerg Med* 1997; 29: 459.

Risk Factors for Cardiac Syncope	
Risk factor	*Odds ratio*[1]
Abnormal EKG (any abnormality except non-specific ST-T waves)	3.2
History of vent. arrhythmia	4.8
History of congestive failure	3.1
Age > 45 years	3.2

[1] Odds ratio is roughly equivalent to increased risk of death compared to patients with syncope, but without that particular risk factor.

Valvular Heart Disease

Disorder	Murmur	Clinical features
Aortic regurgitation	high-pitched, blowing diastolic, after S2	dyspnea, fatigue, pulmonary edema, chest pain, wide pulse pressure
Aortic stenosis (AS)	harsh, systolic ejection right 2nd IC space to carotids, paradoxical S2 split, S3/S4 common	dyspnea (earliest symptom), syncope, angina, narrow pulse pressure, EKG with LVH, or (RBBB or LBBB in 10%)
Idiopathic Hypertrophic, Subaortic Stenosis (IHSS)	crescendo-decrescendo harsh systolic at apex or left sternal border.	similar to AS symptoms with earlier age onset (30-40 years), louder with exercise, and softer with squatting
Mitral regurgitation (Acute)	harsh apical systolic, crescendo-decrescendo starts at S1 + ends before S2, S3+S4	dyspnea, tachycardia, and acute pulmonary edema, angina (may be masked by dyspnea), shock. EKG without left atrial or vent. hypertrophy
Mitral regurgitation (Chronic)	high pitched apical holosystolic radiates to axilla, S3 followed by short diastolic rumble	1st exertional dyspnea, atrial fib., emboli (20%), late parasternal lift (heave). EKG usually shows left atrial and ventricular hypertrophy
Mitral stenosis	mid-diastolic apical, crescendos into S2, loud opening snap, loud S1	exertional dyspnea, orthopnea, hemoptysis, PACs, atrial fibrillation (40%), emboli (14%) , normal to low BP
Tricuspid regurgitation	high-pitched, pansystolic, at 4th para-sternal space	orthopnea, right sided failure (JVD), edema, large liver/spleen, ascites), EKG shows RBBB, or atrial fib.

Electrolyte Disorders

CALCIUM

Hypocalcemia - Total calcium < 8.5 mg/dl or ionized Ca^{+2} < 2.0 mEq/L (1.0 mmol/L)
Hypercalcemia - Total calcium > 10.5 mg/dl or ionized Ca^{+2} > 2.7 mEq/L (1.3 mmol/L)
Hypoalbuminemia – a serum albumin ↓of 1 g/dl will↓ total serum Ca^{+2} 0.8 mg/dl

Hypocalcemia – Clinical Features

Symptoms	Physical Findings	Electrocardiogram
Paresthesias, fatigue	Hyperactive reflexes	• Prolonged QT
Seizures, tetany	Chvostek(C)/Trousseau(T) signs[1]	(esp. Ca^{+2} < 6.0 mg/dl)
Vomiting, weakness	Low blood pressure	• Bradycardia,
Laryngospasm	Congestive heart failure	• Arrhythmias

[1]C–muscle twitch if tap facial nerve, T–carpal spasm after forearm BP cuff X 3 min

Hypocalcemia Evaluation

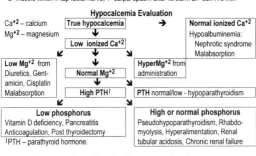

Ca^{+2} – calcium
Mg^{+2} – magnesium

True hypocalcemia → Normal ionized Ca^{+2}
Hypoalbuminemia:
Nephrotic syndrome
Malabsorption

↓

Low ionized Ca^{+2}

↓

Low Mg^{+2} from
Diuretics, Gentamicin, Cisplatin
Malabsorption

Normal Mg^{+2} ← HyperMg^{+2} from administration

↓

High PTH[1] → PTH normal/low - hypoparathyroidism

Low phosphorus
Vitamin D deficiency, Pancreatitis
Anticoagulation, Post thyroidectomy

High or normal phosphorus
Pseudohypoparathyroidism, Rhabdomyolysis, Hyperalimentation, Renal tubular acidosis, Chronic renal failure

[1]PTH – parathyroid hormone.

Drugs That Can Cause Hypocalcemia

• Cimetidine	• Glucagon	• Phosphates
• Cisplatin	• Glucocorticoids	• Protamine
• Citrate (transfusion)	• Heparin	• Norepinephrine
• Dilantin, phenobarbital	• Loop diuretics (*Lasix*)	• Sodium nitroprusside
• Gentamicin, Tobramycin	• Magnesium sulfate	• Theophylline

Hypocalcemia Treatment

Drug	Preparation	Drug Dose[1]
Ca gluconate	10% solution – 93 mg/ 10 ml	10-20 ml IV over 3-5 minutes
Ca chloride	10% solution – 273 mg/ 10ml	5 ml in 50 ml D5W IV over 10 min

[1] IV calcium may cause hypotension, tissue necrosis, bradycardia or digoxin toxicity.
Consider administration via central line, if possible to prevent extravasation risk.

Hypercalcemia – Clinical Features

General	• Weakness, polydipsia, dehydration
Neurologic	• Confusion, irritability, hyporeflexia, headache
Skeletal	• Bone pain, fractures
Cardiac	• Hypertension, QT shortening, wide T wave, arrhythmias
GI	• Anorexia, weight loss, constipation, ulcer, pancreatitis
Renal	• Polyuria, renal insufficiency, nephrolithiasis

Hypercalcemia Evaluation

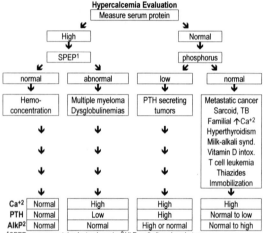

	normal	abnormal	low	normal
Measure serum protein	High → SPEP[1]		Normal → phosphorus	
	Hemo-concentration	Multiple myeloma Dysglobulinemias	PTH secreting tumors	Metastatic cancer Sarcoid, TB Familial ↑Ca^{+2} Hyperthyroidism Milk-alkali synd. Vitamin D intox. T cell leukemia Thiazides Immobilization
Ca^{+2}	Normal	High	High	High
PTH	Normal	Low	High	Normal to low
AlkP[2]	Normal	Normal	High or normal	Normal to high

[1]SPEP – serum protein electrophoresis; [2]AlkP – alkaline phosphatase

Hypercalcemia Management

- IV normal saline 1-2 Liters bolus, then 200-500 ml/hour
- Furosemide (*Lasix*) 10-40 mg IV q 2-4 h to keep urine output 200-300 ml/h
- Consider central line, and watch closely for signs of heart failure or overload
- Follow urine magnesium (Mg), and potassium (K$^+$) losses, replacing prn or empirically administering 15 mg Mg/hour and 10-30 mEq K$^+$/hour
- Consider dialysis with calcium free dialysate if renal failure
- EDTA at 10-50 mg/kg IV over 4 hours ONLY if life threatening features
- Other adjuncts: calcitonin, mithramycin, diphosphonates, galium, steroids

MAGNESIUM

Hypomagnesemia (<1.5 mEq/L):Due to alcohol, diuretics, aminoglycosides, malnourished. Irritable muscle, tetany, seizures. Treat: $MgSO_4$ 5-10 mg/kg IV over 20 min.

Hypermagnesemia (>2.2 mEq/L) Due to renal failure, excess maternal Mg supplement, or overuse of Mg-containing medicine. Clinical features: weakness, hyporeflexia, paralysis, and EKG with AV block and QT prolongation. Treat: Ca chloride (10%) 20 mg/kg IV.

POTASSIUM

Acute decreases in pH will increase K^+ (a $\downarrow$pH of 0.1 will $\uparrow K^+$ 0.3-1.3 mEq/L).

Causes of Hypokalemia	
• Decreased K^+ intake • Intracellular shift (normal stores): alkalemia, insulin, pseudohypokalemia of leukemia, familial hypokalemic periodic paralysis (HPP).	• Increased excretion: diuretics, hyperaldosteronism, penicillins (exchange Na^+/K^+), sweating, diarrhea (colonic fluid has high K^+), vomiting (compensation for metabolic alkalosis)

Hypokalemia Evaluation

Measure blood pH (pH), serum CO_2, and Cl^-

$\downarrow CO_2$, $\uparrow Cl^-$			normal CO_2, Cl^-	$\uparrow CO_2$, $\downarrow Cl^-$
pH < 7.35 Met acidosis[1]	pH > 7.45 Resp alkalosis[2]	pH 7.35-7.45 Met. Acidosis Resp alkalosis	Normal pH	pH > 7.45 Met. alkalosis
RTA[3] 1 or 2	Diarrhea	Cirrhosis Sepsis Salicylates	Hypokalemic periodic paralysis	Diuretics,$\downarrow$Mg Vomiting Laxative abuse Hyperaldosteronism Licorice abuse
Urine pH > 6.5 Urine K^+ > 30 mM/d	Urine pH < 5.3 Urine K^+ < 30 mM/d			

[1]Metabolic acidosis, [2]Respiratory alkalosis, [3]Renal tubular acidosis

Clinical Features of Hypokalemia	Treatment of Hypokalemia
• Lethargy, confusion weakness • Areflexia, difficult respirations • Autonomic instability, Low BP	• Ensure good urine output first • If mild, replace orally only • Parenteral K^+ if severe hypokalemia (e.g. cardiac, or neuromuscular symptoms or DKA).
EKG findings in Hypokalemia	
• $K^+ \leq 3.0$ mEq/L: low voltage QRS, flat T's, $\downarrow$ST, prominent P & U wave • $K^+ \leq 2.5$ mEq/L: prominent U waves • $K^+ \leq 2.0$ mEq/L: widened QRS	• Administer K^+ at ≤ 10 mEq/h using ≤ 40 mEq/L while on cardiac monitor. • 40 mEq raises serum K^+ by 1 mEq/L

Hyperkalemia

Causes of Hyperkalemia

• *Pseudohyperkalemia* due to blood sampling or hemolysis. • *Exogenous*: blood, salt substitutes, potassium containing drugs (e.g. penicillin derivatives), acute digoxin toxicity, β blockers, succinylcholine.	• *Endogenous* – acidemia, trauma, burns, rhabdomyolysis, DIC, sickle cell crisis, GI bleed, chemotherapy (destroying tumor mass), mineralo-corticoid deficiency), congenital defects (21 hydroxylase deficiency)

Hyperkalemia Evaluation

Measure CO_2 and Cl^-

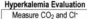

Low serum CO_2	Normal CO_2 and Cl^-
Serum pH < 7.35 Metabolic acidosis	Serum pH 7.35-7.45
• Renal failure • Hypoaldosteronism (e.g. Addison's) • Diabetic Ketoacidosis	• Insulin deficiency & hyperglycemia • Pseudohyperkalemia (e.g. high WBC or high platelets)

Clinical Features of Hyperkalemia	Treatment of Hyperkalemia
• Paresthesias, weakness • Ascending paralysis sparing head, trunk, and respiration.	• Calcium gluconate[1] (10%)–10 ml IV over 2-5 min, may repeat X 2 **OR** • $CaCl_2$[1] (10%) 1 amp IV over 5 min • $NaHCO_3$[2] 50 mEq (1 amp) IV, repeat In 15 min, then 2 amps in 1L D5W IV

EKG in Hyperkalemia (K+ in mEq/L)	
K+	**EKG findings**
> 5.5-6	Peaked T waves
> 6-6.5	↑ PR and QT intervals
> 6.5-7	↓ P, ↓ ST segments
> 7-7.5	↑intraventricular conduction
> 7.5-8	↑ QRS, ST&T waves merge
> 10.0	sine wave appearance

Treatment of Hyperkalemia (continued):
• Glucose/Insulin – 10 units regular insulin IV + 1 amp D_{50} IV, then 10-20 units regular insulin in 500 ml D10W IV over 1 h if needed
• Albuterol nebulizer 5 mg, may repeat
• Furosemide 40 mg IV
• Kayexalate 20 g PO or 50 g PR
• Dialysis

[1] Contraindicated if digoxin toxicity

[2] Relatively contraindication if fluid overload

SODIUM

FE_{Na} = fraction of Na^+ in urine filtered by the glomerulus and not reabsorbed.

FE_{Na} = 100 x (urine Na^+/plasma Na^+) ÷ (urine creatinine/plasma creatinine)

Hyponatremia

Na^+ = falsely ↓ 1.6 mEq/L for each 100 mg/dL ↑ in glucose over 100 mg/dL.

Clinical Features of Hyponatremia	
• Lethargy, apathy	• Cerebral edema
• Depressed reflexes, muscle cramps	• Seizures
• Pseudobulbar palsies	• Hypothermia

Hyponatremia Evaluation

Deficit body Na^+ > deficit body water		Excess total body water (no edema)	Excess total body water > excess Na^+ (edema)	
Renal losses: diuretics, mineralocorticoid deficiency, salt losing nephritis, bicarbonaturia, ketonuria, osmotic diuresis	*Extrarenal loss:* vomit, diarrhea, 3rd space fluids, pancreatitis, peritonitis, traumatized muscle	Glucocorticoid deficiency, low thyroid, pain, emotional stress, drugs, (SIADH - U_{osm} usually > S_{osm})	Nephrotic syndrome, cirrhosis, CHF	Acute and chronic renal failure

(Obtain urine Na^+, urine creatinine, urine osmolality, and serum osmolality)

Na^+>20 mEq/L ↑FE_{Na}, ↓ SG[1] U_{osm}[3] varies	Na^+<10 mEq/L ↓FE_{Na}, ↑ SG[1] U_{osm}[3] > 800	Na^+>20 mEq/L Nl[2] FE_{Na}, ↑ SG[1] U_{osm}[3] varies	Na^+<10 mEq/L ↓FE_{Na}, ↑ SG[1] high U_{osm}[3]	Na^+>20 mEq/L ↑FE_{Na}, ↓ SG[1] U_{osm}[3] varies
Management				
Isotonic saline	Isotonic saline	Water restrict	Water restrict	Water restrict

[1] SG - specific gravity, [2] Nl- normal, [3] U_{osm} - urine osmalality, [4] S_{osm} -serum osmolality

Hypertonic Saline Administration (3%NaCl – 513 mEq/L)

Indication • Severe ↓ Na^+ with serious CNS manifestations (e.g. seizures)

Goal • Only ↑Na^+ to 120-125 mEq/L acutely,& maximum of 20 mEq/L/24h

Formula • **Na^+ deficit** = weight (kg) X 0.6 X (desired Na^+[~125] – known Na^+)
 • **Infusion rate (ml/hour)** that will ↑Na^+ 1 mEq/L/hour
 = (weight [kg] X 0.6) ÷ (0.513 mEq/L X 1 hour)

Rate • 2-4 mEq/L/hour - if active seizing, or ↑ intracranial pressure over 1 hour or until seizing stops, then ↓ rate to 1-2 mEq/L/hour
 • 1-2 mEq/L/hour - if obtunded, or other neurologic symptoms

Adjuncts • Furosemide (*Lasix*) – 40 mg IV; remember to check Na^+ q 2 hours

Am J Med 1997; 102: 67.

Hypernatremia

Clinical Features of Hypernatremia	
• Lethargy, irritability, coma • Seizures • Spasticity, hyperreflexia	• Doughy skin • Late preservation of intravascular volume (and vital signs)

Hypernatremia Etiology, Diagnosis and Management

Na$^+$ + H$_2$O loss with low total body Na$^+$		H$_2$O loss with normal total body Na$^+$		Excess Na$^+$ with increased total body Na$^+$
Renal losses osmotic diuresis (mannitol, glucose, urea)	Extrarenal loss excess sweat, diarrhea	Renal loss diabetes insipidus (nephrogenic, central) Serum osm > 295 mosm/L, Serum Na+ > 145 mEq/L, U$_{osm}$ < 150 mosm/L	Extrarenal loss Respiratory and skin loss	Primary hyper-aldosteronism, Cushing's syn-drome, hyper-tonic dialysis, hypertonic Na$^+$ bicarbonate, NaCl tablets

Diagnosis

BUN normal,↑ U Na$^+$>20 mEq/L, U$_{osm}$ hypotonic	BUN ↑ U Na$^+$<10 mEq/L, U$_{osm}$ > 600-800 mosm/L	BUN ± normal U Na$^+$ varies U$_{osm}$ often < 100-150 mosm/L in central DI	BUN ↑ U Na$^+$ varies U$_{osm}$ > 600-800 mOsm/L	BUN ± normal U Na$^+$>20 mEq/L U$_{osm}$ isotonic or hypertonic

Management

Hypotonic saline	Hypotonic saline	Water replacement D$_5$W	Water replace-ment D$_5$W	Diuretic+H$_2$O re-placement D$_5$W

[1] U-urine, U$_{osm}$ – urine osmolality

Management of Hypernatremia

- Correct hypernatremia slowly over 48 to 72 hours. Overvigorous rehydration can cause cerebral edema, seizures, coma, or death. Lower Na$^+$ no faster than 1-2 mEq/L/hour.
- With endogenous Na$^+$ overload, treatment consists of salt restriction and correction of the primary underlying disorder. If there is excess exogenous mineralocorticoid, restrict salt and modify replacement therapy.

Endocrine Disorders

Adrenal Insufficiency

Clinical Features		Adrenal Crisis Therapy
Weakness	99%	• 1-2 Liters NS IV with further IV fluids as needed
↑pigment	92%	• Correct electrolyte abnormalities
Weight loss	97%	• Hydrocortisone (*Solu-Cortef*) 200 mg IV, + 100 mg q8h
Vomiting	70%	• If possible draw & store blood for steroid level analysis
Anorexia	98%	• Consider broad spectrum antibiotics (e.g. ceftriaxone 1-2 g IV) if suspicion of sepsis
BP < 110/70	85%	• Perform rapid bedside check of blood sugar
Abdominal		• Treat underling precipitants (e.g. sepsis, hypothermia,
Pain	34%	MI, ↓glucose, bleeding, trauma, remove medications
Salt craving	22%	that ↓cortisone: morphine,chlorpromazine,barbiturates)
Diarrhea	20%	

Diabetes Mellitus

INSULIN	Preparation	Onset (h)	Peak (h)	Duration (h)
Rapid acting	Regular	0.5-1	2.5-5	6-8
	Humalog	0-0.25	0.5-1.5	3-4
Intermediate acting	NPH	1-1.5	4-12	24
	Lente	1-2.5	7-15	24
Long acting	Ultralente	4-8	10-30	> 36

Humulin + Novolin 70/30, 50/50 preparations = %NPH/%regular insulin.

Oral Hypoglycemic Medications

	Dose in mg (max daily dose)	Frequency	Onset (hours)	Duration (hours)
1st generation sulfonylureas				
acetohexamide (*Dymelor*)	250, 500 (1500)	qd/bid	1	12-24
chlorpropamide (*Diabenase*)	100, 250 (750)	qd	1	up to 60
tolazamide (*Tolinase*)	100, 250, 500 (1000)	qd	4-6	12-24
tolbutamide (*Orinase*)	500, 1000 (3000)	bid/tid	1	6-12
2nd generation sulfonylureas				
glimipride (*Amaryl*)	1, 2, 4 (8)	qd	1	24
glipizide (*Glucotrol*)	5, 10 (40)	bid/qd	1-1.5	10-16
glyburide (*Diabeta, Micronase*)	1.25, 2.5, 5 (20)	qd	2-4	24
glyburide-micronized (*Glynase*)	1.5, 3, 6 (12)	qd	1	18-24
Non-sulfonylureas				
acarbose (*Precose, Prandase*)[1]	25,50,100 (150-300)	tid (at meal)	0.5	1-3
metformin HCl (*Glucophage*)[2]	500, 850 (2550)	qd/bid/tid	1-4	18-24
migitol (*Glyset*)[1]	25, 50, 100 (300)	tid (at meal)	0.5	1-3
repaglinide (*Prandin*)	0.5, 1, 2 (16)	tid		
troglitazone (*Rezulin*)	200, 400 (600)	qd	2-3	16-34

[1] acts locally by blocking intestinal carbohydrate absorption [2] can cause lactic acidosis, & contrast induced renal failure, must stop use for 24 h before contrast administration

Diabetic Ketoacidosis (DKA)

Laboratory diagnosis of DKA	Precipitants of DKA	
• Blood glucose > 300 mg/dl	• Recent change in insulin dose	40%
• Serum bicarbonate < 15 mEq/L in the absence of chronic renal failure	• Infection	40%
• Serum acetone level > 2:1 dilution	• Noncompliance (diet or meds)	23%
• Arterial pH < 7.30 in 1st 24 hours	• Trauma, injury, and stroke	10%
	• No prior diabetes	20%

Am J Epidemiol 1983; 117: 551.

Management

- Apply cardiac monitor and administer O_2 if altered mental status or shock.
- Obtain labs and assess for DKA precipitants or complications.
- Fluid & electrolyte deficits should generally be replaced over the 1st 24-48 hours.
- <u>IV fluids</u> – IV NS until hypotension, and orthostasis resolve and urine output is ≥ 1 ml/kg/hour. Then administer ½ NS at 500 ml/hour.
- <u>Insulin</u> – 10 units (U) regular insulin IV, then 5-10 U/h IV. Once blood glucose is < 300 mg/dl, add D5 (e.g. D5½ NS) to fluids and↓ insulin dose to 2-4 U/hour. Change to SC regular insulin once bicarbonate > 15 mEq/L and no anion gap.
- <u>Replace potassium</u> (1st verify adequate urine output) and phosphate. If initial K+ is normal or low, add 10-40 mEq K+/L to IV fluids. Replace K+ with ~ 50/50 mix of KCL and K_3PO_4. Check glucose q h until < 300 mg/dl, & electrolytes q 2-4 h.
- <u>Bicarbonate</u> – primarily indicated for hyperkalemia management, if needed.

Hyperosmolar Hyperglycemic Nonketotic Coma (HHNC)

Diagnosis of HHNC	Etiology/Precipitants of HHNC	
• Plasma osmolarity > 350 mOsm/L	Renal failure	Pancreatitis
• Glucose > 600 mg/dl	Pneumonia, Sepsis	Burn
• No ketosis (lactic acidosis ± present)	GI bleed	Heat stroke
• 50-65% have no history of diabetes	MI	Dialysis
• ↑ BUN with BUN/Cr ratio > 30	CNS bleed/stroke	Recent surgery
• ↑ CK due to rhabdomyolysis	Pulmonary emboli	Medicines[1]

[1]Thiazides, Ca^{+2} channel blocker, steroids, *Dilantin*, *Inderal*, *Hygroton*, *Lasix*, *Tagamet*, loxapine.

History		Physical Exam	
Fever	Polydipsia	↓consciousness	Hemiparesis
Thirst	Confusion	Tachycardia, ↓BP	Myoclonus
Polyuria or	Seizures (focal)	Fever	Quadriplegia
Oliguria	Hallucinations	Focal seizure	Nystagmus

Hyperosmolar Hyperglycemic Nonketotic Coma *continued....*

Treatment

- Admit all patients to the ICU, and consider placement of central line.
- Obtain electrolytes, CK, UA, CXR, EKG, cultures, ± cranial CT and spinal tap.
- <u>Fluids</u>- mean fluid deficit is 9 L. Start IV NS until BP & urine output OK. Then, change to ½NS & replace 50% of deficit over 12 h, & 50% over next 12-24 h.
- <u>Add dextrose</u> (D5½NS) once glucose falls ≤ 300 mg/dl.
- <u>Replace potassium</u> (5-10 mEq per h) when level available, and OK urine output.
- <u>Insulin</u> may be unnecessary. Consider single 0.1 U/kg IV dose with 0.05 U/kg/hr IV until glucose is 300 mg/dl.
- Consider empiric phosphate repletion, subcutaneous heparin and broad-spectrum prophylactic antibiotics to treat and prevent potential complications.

Hypoglycemia
Etiology

- *Fasting hypoglycemia* from glucose. Symptoms begin 4-6 h after meal. (1) overuse (drugs - p 29, insulin, sepsis, tumors, starvation, exercise) or (2) underproduction (alcohol, β blockers, salicylate, hormone deficiency, liver or renal failure, enzyme defects, or substrate defects as in malnutrition).
- *Reactive hypoglycemia* begins within 1-2 h of meal and is due to impaired GI motility, impaired glucose tolerance (?early diabetes), or enzyme defect.

Clinical features

- Sympathetic response: tachycardia, hunger, tremors, or sweating. These may be absent in diabetics, alcoholics, and those on β blockers.
- Neuronal dysfunction: headache, coma, seizures, focal deficits.

Treatment

- Glucose 1 amp (50 ml) of $D_{50}W$ IV (↑glucose ~ 150 mg/dl) or glucagon 1 mg IM/SC if no IV. Then IV D_5NS or $D_{10}NS$ to maintain normal blood glucose.
- Hydrocortisone (*Solu-Cortef*) 100 mg IV if possible adrenal insufficiency.
- Thiamine 100 mg IV or IM if malnourished.
- Diazoxide (*Hyperstat*) 1-2 mg/kg IV if unable to control with IV glucose.
- Admit all intentional oral hypoglycemic and insulin overdoses.
- If mild unintentional insulin overdose, administer D50 or oral glucose, feed meal, observe for a short time period and discharge.
- If short acting 2nd generation sulfonylurea, no recurrent symptoms over 6-8 h, and charcoal given, some recommend discharge. Otherwise admit all oral hypoglycemic overdoses.

Hyperthyroidism/Thyroid Storm

Underlying Thyroid Disease	Precipitants of Thyroid Storm	
• Grave's disease (most common)	Infection (#1)	Iodine therapy/dye
• Toxic nodular goiter	Pulmonary embolus	Stroke
• Toxic adenoma	DKA, or HHNC	Surgery
• Factitious thyrotoxicosis	Thyroid hormone	Childbirth
• Excess TSH	excess	D&C

Clinical Features of Thyroid Storm (Thyrotoxicosis)		
Hyperkinesis	Temperature > 101 F	Psychosis, apathy, coma
Palpable goiter	↑HR + ↑pulse pressure	Tremor, hyperreflexia
Proptosis, lid lag	Arrhythmia (new onset)[2]	Diarrhea, weight loss
Exophthalmos, palsy[1]	Palpitations, dyspnea	Jaundice

[1]Palsy of extraocular muscles, [2]Atrial fibrillation/flutter which may be refractory to digoxin

Laboratory Features of Thyrotoxicosis[1]	• ↑freeT_4, ↑T_3, ↓TSH • ↑T_4RIA, ↑FT_4I	• ↑glucose,↑Ca^{+2},↓Hb, ↑WBC,↓cholesterol

[1]Laboratory tests can diagnose hyperthyroidism, but thyrotoxicosis is a clinical diagnosis.

Treatment

- Supportive care, O_2, bedside glucose check, fever control (avoid aspirin) and treat precipitants.
- Inhibit thyroid hormone synthesis: Propylthiouracil (PTU) 900-1200 mg PO on day 1, then 300-600 mg/d PO X 3-6 weeks. PTU inhibits conversion of T_4 to T_3.
- Inhibit thyroid hormone release: K^+ iodide as Lugol's solution (8 mg iodide/drop) - 1 ml or 20 drops PO q 8 h. OR SSKI (40 mg iodide/drop) 2-10 drops PO daily. OR Na^+ iodide 1 g IV q 8-12 hours (give over 30 min). Caution: Administer iodide ≥ 1 h after anti-thyroid medications to prevent use in hormone synthesis.
- Blockade of peripheral effects: Consider Propanolol 1 mg slowly IV q 15 min (Max 10 mg) prn to reduce sympathetic hyperactivity and conversion of T_4 to T_3. Begin propanolol 20-120 mg PO q 4-6 hours when symptoms improve.
- Inhibit conversion of T4 to T3: hydrocortisone (Solu-Cortef) 100 mg IV q 8h.

Apathetic Thyrotoxicosis

A rare form of thyrotoxicosis usually occurring in the elderly.

Clinical Features		Management
• Mean age > 60 years	• Weak proximal muscles	Treat as thyro-
• Lethargy, ↓ mentation	• Mean weight loss > 40 lb.	toxicosis but use
• No Grave's eye signs	• Atrial fibrillation (in 75%)	lower doses &
• Smaller goiter	• Congestive heart failure	slower rates as
• Depression/apathy	• Atrial fibrillation/CHF may	side effects are
	be refractory to treatment	greater in elderly.

Hypothyroidism/Myxedema Coma

Precipitants of Myxedema Coma		Lab tests
Pneumonia, GI bleed	*Drugs*	Serum TSH > 60 µU/ml
CHF, cold exposure	Phenothiazines,	↓ total & free T4
Stroke, trauma, ↓glucose	narcotics, sedatives,	↓ or ↔ total & free T3
↓pO$_2$,↑pCO$_2$, ↓Na$^+$	phenytoin, propranolol	

Clinical Features of Myxedema Coma	
Vitals	• Temperature is often < 90 F, 50% have BP < 100/60
Cardiac	• ↓HR, heart block, low voltage, ST-T changes, ↑Q-T, effusion
Pulmonary	• Hypoventilation, ↑pCO$_2$, ↓O$_2$, pleural effusions
Metabolic	• Hyponatremia, hypoglycemia
Neurologic	• Coma, seizures, tremors, ataxia, nystagmus, psychiatric disturbances. Depressed or "hung up" reflexes
GI/GU	• Ileus, ascites, fecal impaction, megacolon, urinary retention
Skin	• Alopecia, loss of lateral 1/3 eyebrows, nonpitting puffiness around eyes, hands, and pretibial region of legs
ENT	• Tongue enlarges, voice deepens and becomes hoarse

Treatment

- Administer O$_2$, rewarm and treat cause (e.g. infection, ↓ glucose).
- Thyroxine – 400-500 µg slow IV on day 1, + 50-100 µg IV q day. **CAUTION** IV thyroxine may cause cardiac arrest. Reduce dose if cardiac ischemia or arrhythmias. Some experts recommend no IV thyroxine for 3-7 days after day 1.
- Start oral thyroxine 100-200 µg PO q day when possible.
- Hydrocortisone (*Solu-Cortef*) 100 mg IV q 8h.

Environmental Disorders

Scuba Diving Injuries (Dysbarism)

<u>Dysbaric air embolism (DAE)</u>: gas bubbles enter circulation through ruptured pulmonary veins causing symptoms within 10 minutes of surfacing. Symptoms: cardiac arrest, seizure, cardiac ischemia, stroke, and asymmetric multiplegias.

<u>Decompression sickness (DCS)</u>: formation of gas bubbles in blood and body tissues following ↓ in ambient pressure. ↑ risk with old age, obesity, dehydration, alcohol use, exercise, unpressurized flight after dive. Symptoms occur 10 min-6 h (rarely delayed 24-48 h) after ascent and are due to bubbles causing vascular occlusion. <u>Type I DCS</u> involves lymphatics, skin (mottled rash, itching), musculoskeletal (periarticular joint pain worse with movement) esp. shoulders and elbows.

Diving Injuries continued ...

<u>Type II DCS</u> causes neurologic disruption with spinal cord involvement (low thoracic, lumbar, and sacral primarily) with paraplegia, and bladder dysfunction. Pulmonary involvement with pain, dyspnea, and edema may occur.

DCS and DAE Management

- Administer 100% Oxygen and IV NS unless contraindicated.
- Exclude treatable injuries (e.g. pneumothorax).
- Do not place in Trendelenberg. This worsens CNS edema and dyspnea.
- Transport to nearest hyperbaric recompression chamber. If uncertain where nearest facility is call **(919) 684-8111)**. Must fly at low altitude < 1000 feet or use aircraft that can pressurize to 1 atmosphere (ATA).

High Altitude Syndromes

Acute Mountain Sickness – AMS

- *Risk factors*: rapid ascent, high sleeping altitudes, 25% > 6900 feet (2000 meters), low vital capacity, low hypoxic ventilatory response (COPD).
- *Clinical Features*: Early on lightheadedness and breathlessness, in 1-24 h, hangover (headache, anorexia, vomiting, irritability, sleepiness), and later dyspnea, oliguria, high altitude cerebral or pulmonary edema (20% have local rales) occurs with retinal hemorrhages > 5000 meters.
- *Prevention*: Diamox or Decadron 24 h (see above) preascent + 2 d after ascent.

Treatment - AMS

1. Stop ascent or descend if worsening, and O_2 0.5-1 L/min at night
2. Acetazolamide (*Diamox*) 125-250 mg PO bid to speed acclimatization
3. Dexamethasone (*Decadron*) 4 mg PO q6h
4. Hyperbaric oxygen therapy (e.g. hyperbaric bag)

High Altitude Cerebral Edema - HACE

Progressive neurologic deterioration in someone with HAPE or AMS.
Clinical Features: altered mental status, ataxia, stupor and coma if untreated. Headache and vomiting are not always present. Focal deficits may occur.

Treatment

1. Immediate descent or evacuation, supplemental O_2
2. Dexamethasone (*Decadron*) 8 mg PO, IM, or IV then 4 mg q 6h
3. Acetazolamide (*Diamox*) 125 mg PO bid may be useful as an adjunct
4. If coma, intubation and hyperventilation (patients already have low pCO_2, and too much hyperventilation can lead to cerebral ischemia)
5. Furosemide (*Lasix*) 40-80 mg IV (avoid dehydration, and hypotension)
6. Hyperbaric oxygen therapy (e.g. hyperbaric bag)

High Altitude Pulmonary Edema - HAPE

- *Risk factors*: male sex, child, erection, rapid ascent, cold, excess salt, sleeping medications, prior HAPE/AMS. HAPE is a noncardiogenic edema due to exaggerated pulmonary pressor response to hypoxia.
- *Clinical Features*: initially dry cough, poor exercise, local rales, and later development of tachycardia, tachypnea, dyspnea, cyanosis, generalized rales, and coma. Symptoms of AMS need not be present. A right ventricular heave may be noted. ECG may show right axis deviation, and right ventricular strain.

Treatment

1. Immediate descent (with minimal exertion by victim), warming, supplemental O_2
2. Hyperbaric therapy, morphine 2-5 mg IV, furosemide (*Lasix*) 40-80 mg IV
3. Continuous positive airway pressure (CPAP) or expiratory positive airway pressure (EPAP) mask (can ↑ O_2 saturation ~ 20%),
4. Nifedipine (*Procardia*) 10 mg PO reduces pulmonary artery pressure by 30-50% and increases arterial O_2 saturation. Nifedipine (extended release) 30 mg PO q8h while ascending may prophylax against development of HAPE.

Hyperthermia and Hypothermia

Minor Heat Illness

- <u>Heat Syncope</u>: Postural hypotension from vasodilation, volume depletion, and ↓ vascular tone. Rehydrate, remove from heat, and evaluate for serious disease.
- <u>Heat cramps</u>: Painful, contractions of calves, thigh, or shoulders in those who are sweating liberally and drinking hypotonic solutions (e.g. water). Replace fluids: 0.1-0.2% oral solution or IV NS rehydration. Do not use salt tablets.
- <u>Heat Exhaustion</u>: Salt and water depletion causing orthostasis, and hyperthermia (usually < 104F). Mental status, and neurologic exam are normal. Lab: high hematocrit, high sodium, or high BUN. Treat with NS 1-2 Liters IV.

Heatstroke

Clinical Features	Risk Factors
• Hyperpyrexia (>104-105.8F/40-41C)	• Old age, skin disorders, obesity

• Central nervous system dysfunction (seizures, altered mentation, plantar responses, hemiplegia, ataxia)	• Drugs
	  - amphetamines
	  - anticholinergics

• Loss of sweating (variably present)	- antihypertensive agents
• ↓ Na, ↓ Ca, ↓ phosphate, ↓ or ↑ K	- sympathomimetics (e.g. cocaine)
• Rhabdomyolysis, renal or liver failure	- phenothiazines

Management of Heatstroke

- Administer oxygen, protect airway if comatose or seizing. Check blood glucose.
- Measure temperature with continuous rectal probe accurate at high levels.
- Begin IV NS cautiously as pulmonary edema is common and mean fluid requirement is only 1.2 L in first 4 hours. Consider central line pressures as guide.
- Immediate cooling by: (1) *evaporation*: Spray with tepid water and direct fan at patient (0.1 - 0.3C/min temp. drop). For shivering, IV lorazepam 1-3 mg IV. (2) *ice water (or 60F) tub immersion*: (*controversial*) (temp. drop ~ 0.16C/min). (3) *Ice packs*, *cooling blankets*, *peritoneal dialysis*, *gastric lavage* with cold water are slow or unproven. (4) Avoid aspirin (hyperpyrexia). Avoid repeated Tylenol doses (possible liver damage and ineffective in heatstroke).
- Stop above measures at temperature of 102-104 to avoid over-correction.
- Place Foley catheter to monitor urine output (see rhabdomyolysis below).
- Obtain CBC, electrolytes, renal function, glucose, liver enzymes, LDH/CK, PT, and PTT, arterial blood gas, and fibrin degradation products. ECG and CXR.
- Exclude other fever cause: infection, malignant hyperthermia, thyroid, drugs, etc

Other Heat Related Disorders

- **Malignant hyperthermia (MH)**: Autosomal dominant disorder causing fever, & rigid muscles after anesthetics or succinylcholine is administered. *Treatment*: Stop agent, lower temperature as in heatstroke (avoid phenothiazines), give dantrolene 2-3 mg/kg IV q 6 hours (max 10 mg/kg/day).
- **Neuroleptic Malignant Syndrome:** Similar to MH with fever, muscle rigidity, and altered mentation, but due to anticholinergics (e.g. phenothiazines). *Treatment:* Stop agent, treat heatstroke (avoid phenothiazines) and administer benzodiazepines IV (e.g. lorazepam), dantrolene 2-3 mg/kg IV (max 10 mg/kg) and bromocriptine 2.5-10 mg PO tid.
- **Rhabdomyolysis:** Syndrome with release of contents into circulation due to tissue hypoxia, direct injury, exercise, enzyme defects, metabolic disease (DKA, ↓ K, ↓ Na, or ↓ phosphate, thyroid), toxins, infections, heatstroke. *Complications[1]*: renal failure,↑K+,↑Ca+2 or↓ Ca+2,↑or↓phosphate,↑ uric acid, compartment syndrome, disseminated intravascular coagulation. *Treatment*: (1) IV NS to keep urine output > 100-200 ml/hr, (2) NaHCO3 ≥ 50 mEq IV to keep urine pH > 6.5, (3) If poor urine output, administer Mannitol – 25-50 g IV,+ 12.5 g to each L of NS, (4) Dialyze if ↑K+ or uremia is present.

[1] R = 0.7 [K+-mEq/L] + 1.1 [Cr-mg/dl] + 0.6 [albumin-g/dl] – 6.6;
  A single retrospective study found that a R ≥ 0.1 had a 41% risk of myoglobinuria induced renal failure, while a R < 0.1 had a 0% risk.   *Medicine* 1982; 3: 141.

HYPOTHERMIA

Severity	Temp. F (C)	Features
Mild	91-95 (33-35)	Maximal shivering + slurred speech at 95F
Moderate	85-90 (29-32)	At 89 – altered mental status, mydriasis, shivering ceases, muscles are rigid, incoordination, bradypnea
Severe	≤ 82 (≤ 28)	Bradycardia in 50%, Osborne waves on EKG, voluntary motion stops, pupils are fixed dilated
	79　(26)	Loss of consciousness, areflexia, no pain response
	77　(25)	No respirations, appear dead, pulmonary edema
	68　(20)	Asystole

Management of Hypothermia
• No vigorous manipulation or active external rewarming unless mild hypothermia
• Evaluate for cause (e.g. sepsis, hypoglycemia, CNS disease, adrenal crisis).
• **Mild hypothermia** (> 32C): Administer humidified warmed O_2. Passive external rewarming and treatment of underlying disease is often only treatment needed.
• **Moderate hypothermia (29-32C):** Use active internal rewarming. Drugs and cardioversion for cardiac arrest are frequently ineffective. Warm humidified O_2, with gastric or peritoneal lavage if < 1C per hour temperature rise. Perform CPR, and advanced life support prn.
• **Severe hypothermia** (≤ 29 C): (1) Warm humidified O_2, and warm IV fluids. (2) If nonarrested, warmed peritoneal dialysis (41C dialysate), or (3) pleural irrigation (41C). (4) If core temperature < 25C consider femoral-femoral bypass. (5) Use open pleural lavage for direct cardiac rewarming if core temperature < 28C after 1 h of bypass in an arrest rhythm. If signs of life, and non-arrested, avoid CPR, and ACLS. If arrested, CPR and ACLS are OK. (6) Use bretylium 5mg/kg for ventricular fibrillation. Do not treat atrial arrhythmias. (7) Treat hypotension with NS 1st. Use pressors cautiously. (8) Consider empiric D_{50}, thiamine 100 mg IV, *Narcan* 2mg IV, + hydrocortisone 100 mg IV.

Snake Bite Envenomation

Grade	Features of Crotalid (Pit viper) envenomation	Antivenin dose
None	± Fang marks, no pain, erythema or systemic symptoms	None
Mild[1]	Fang marks, mild pain/edema, no systemic symptoms	0-5 vials (50 ml)
Moderate	Fang marks, severe pain, moderate edema in 1st 12h, mild symptoms (vomiting, paresthesias), mild coagulopathy (without bleeding)	10 vials (100 ml)
Severe	Fang marks, severe pain/edema, severe symptoms (hypotension, dyspnea), coagulopathy with bleeding	15-20 vials (150-200 ml)

[1]Controversial – some experts recommend no antivenin for mild envenomation.

Prehospital Treatment for Crotalid Envenomation

- Decrease patient movement, and transport to nearest medical facility.
- Immobilize extremity in neutral position below level of heart.
- Incision + drainage and tourniquets are unproven and not recommended.

Emergency Treatment for Crotalid Envenomation

- Perform exam, measure envenomation site, and administer fluids, pressors prn.
- If no signs of envenomation, clean wound, administer tetanus and observe for a minimum of 6 hours. Consider antibiotics (e.g. _Augmentin_ X 5 days).
- If significant envenomation, obtain CBC, electrolytes, renal and liver function tests, PT, PTT, fibrinogen, urinalysis, ECG, and type and cross.
- Perform skin test only if antivenin to be administered: 0.2 ml SC (diluted 1:10 with NS) at a site distant from bite. Observe for signs of allergy for at least 10 minutes after injection. A negative reaction does not entirely exclude allergy.
- Need for antivenin and specific dose is controversial. Prior to administration, obtain consent, expand vascular volume with NS, consider premedication with diphenhydramine 1 mg/kg IV, and dilute antivenin in 50-100 ml for each vial.

Antivenin Administration (see dose above)

- Reconstitute antivenin in a 1:10 solution with NS or D_5W.
- Administer 5-10 ml over 5 min. If no allergy, increase rate so that infusion takes 1-2 hours. If symptoms progress, additional antivenin may be required.
- If allergic reaction and antivenin is necessary, start arterial line, continue to treat with NS ± albumin, methylprednisolone 100 mg IV, and _Benadryl_ 50 mg IV. Hang epinephrine drip in line separate from antivenin (e.g. 0.6mg/kg epi 1:1,000 in 100 ml NS), and maximally dilute antivenin. Begin antivenin slowly. If needed begin epi drip at low dose [1 ml/hr of above mixture = 0.1 µg/kg/min] Once allergic reaction gone, restart antivenin slowly. Contact local poison center.

Elapidae (Coral Snake) Envenomation

This species is found in the southeast US and Arizona. They must bite and chew. Symptoms are primarily systemic and not local: altered mentation, cranial nerve or muscle weakness, respiratory failure. Symptoms may be delayed up to 24 h. Admit all for possible respiratory or neurologic deterioration. All require Coral Snake Antivenin. Dose of antivenin: 3-6 vials administered as crotalidae antivenin. Sonoran (Arizona) coral snake venom is less toxic, no deaths have been reported, and coral snake antivenin is ineffective.

Special Situations

Mojave rattlesnake: May cause muscle weakness, paralysis, or respiratory failure with few local symptoms. Empiric crotalid antivenin is indicated in most instances.
Exotic snakes: Call **(602) 626-6016** for information regarding available anti-venin.
Serum sickness will develop in most receiving > 5 vials of antivenin within 5-20 days causing joint pain, myalgias, and possibly rash. Warn patient and treat with diphenhydramine (*Benadryl*) 25-50 mg PO q4-6 h and prednisone 50 mg PO qd.

Spider Bites

Black Widow Spiders	Features of Black Widow Bites
• Found in all of US, mostly South	• Mild to moderately painful bite,
• Females average 5 cm with legs	• In 1hour, redness, swelling, &
• Only females are toxic	cramping at bite which later spread.
• 1/5 have red hour glass on abdomen	• Abdominal wall pain mimics peritonitis
	• ↓BP, shock, coma, respiratory failure

Management of Black Widow Spider Bites	
• Ca^{+2} gluconate 10%, 10 ml IV	**Indications[1] for Admission/Antivenin**
• Lorazepam (*Ativan*) 1-3 mg IV	• Respiratory or cardiac symptoms
• Consider Antivenin – Dose:	• Pregnancy or > 65 y with symptoms
1-2 vials IV in 50-100 ml NS	• Severe cramping or pain despite
Skin test prior to using	calcium and lorazepam use
Allergy & serum sickness can occur	• History of ↑ BP or cardiac disease

[1]controversial   *Emerg Med Clin North Am* 1992; 269

Brown Recluse Spiders	Management
• Live mostly in southern US, and dark	• Wound care, tetanus
Places. Bites are mild or painless.	• Consider excising if > 2 cm & well-
• At 1st lesions are red and blanch	circumscribed border (usually 2 to 3
• Later a macule, ulcer or blister	weeks after bite)
• Arthralgias, GI upset, DIC, or shock	• ± Dapsone 50-250 mg PO bid
• Hemoglobinuria (renal failure)	• ± Hyperbaric oxygen (controversial)

Marine Envenomation

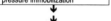 **Puncture Wounds**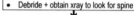

Sea snakes, blue ring octopus cone shells	Starfish, sea urchin, stingrays, catfish weeverfish, scorpionfish

↓ ↓

Lymphatic venous occlusion and pressure immobilization	• Immerse in hot water (45C) X 30-90 min or until pain subsides • Irrigate, after local/regional anesthesia • Debride + obtain xray to look for spine

↓ ↓

Supportive and respiratory care Sea snake antivenin[1,3]	Provide supportive care and administer Stone fish (scorpionfish) antivenin[2,3]

[1] **Sea snakes**. Bites are painless, causing paralysis + muscle necrosis. Administer polyvalent sea snake antivenin (Commonwealth Serum Lab, Australia) within 36 h. If unavailable, Tiger snake and polyvalent *Elapidae* antivenin are effective.

[2] **Stone fish (a type of scorpionfish)**. Venom causes muscle toxicity, with paralysis of cardiac, skeletal, and involuntary muscles. Pain is immediate and intense. The wound is ischemic, cyanotic and may lose tissue. Heat (45C) partially inactivates venom. Follow package insert for antivenin (Commonwealth Serum Labs, Australia).

[3] In US, call **(619) 222-6363** or **(415) 770-7171** for antivenin.

↙ **Marine Exposures Causing Urticaria or Vesicles** ↘

Hydroids, fire coral, jellyfish, anemones	Sponges, bristleworms

↓ ↓

• Apply acetic acid 5%, isopropyl alcohol, 40-70%, or baking soda x 30 min • Remove nematocysts with forceps[1]	Extract spicules, with adhesive tape

  ↓

  Acetic acid 5% or isopropyl alcohol

↓ ↓

• Supportive care for systemic reaction • Antivenin for box jellyfish, *C. flexneri* • Consider systemic steroids	• Topical steroids if mild reaction • Treat for allergic reactions

[1] Do not rinse in fresh water.

Marine Infections

- Organisms causing soft tissue infection: *Aeromonas hydrophilia, B. fragilis, E. coli, Pseudomonas, Salmonella, Vibrio, Staph./Strep.* species, *C. perfringens.*
- Irrigate, debride, explore, and obtain x-rays to exclude foreign bodies
- Antibiotic agents for treating soft tissue infection or prophylaxis:
  <u>Parenteral agents</u> - 3rd generation cephalosporin and/or an aminoglycoside
  <u>Oral agents</u> -*Septra*, tetracycline, cefuroxime, or ciprofloxacin.

Gastrointestinal Bleeding

Upper GI Bleeding

Resuscitation of Upper GI Bleeding	Most Common Diagnoses	
• Administer O$_2$, apply cardiac monitor, insert NG, start NS 2 L IV. Consider transfusion.	Duodenal ulcer	36%
	Gastric ulcer	24%
• Type & cross for 4-6U PRBC's. Obtain CBC, platelets, electrolytes[1], liver function tests, and PT/PTT. Obtain CXR and EKG.	Varices	6%
	Gastritis	6%
	Esophagitis	4%
• Administer FFP if unknown coagulopathy or if PT or PTT > 1.5 X normal.	Mallory Weiss	4%
	Gastroduodenitis	3%
• Administer platelets if level is < 50,000/ml	Other or source not found	17%
	Am J Gastroenterol 1995: 208	

[1] BUN/Cr ratio ≥ 36 indicates a > 95% likelihood the source of bleeding is upper GI.

Evaluation of Upper GI Bleeding

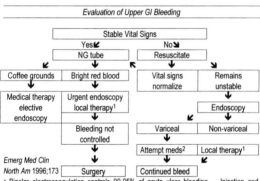

Emerg Med Clin
North Am 1996;173

1 Bipolar electrocoagulation controls 90-95% of acute ulcer bleeding. Injection and sclerotherapy are effective against ulcers and variceal bleeding. Results differ depending upon site and magnitude of bleed.

2 Meds (medications) include (1) *Somatostatin* – lowers portal venous pressure by splanchnic vasoconstriction. <u>Dose</u>: 250 µg IV, then 250 µg/min. OR (2) *Pitressin* - <u>Dose</u>: 0.1-0.9 units/minute IV. Side effects: ↓BP, bowel ischemia, myocardial ischemia, skin necrosis. Nitroglycerin IV (40-400 ug/min) can limit these effects.

Testing gastric aspirate for blood.

- Use gastroccult system to test for blood as hemoccult tests are inaccurate at low pH. Up to 20% with upper GI bleed have negative NG aspirates.
- False positive hemoccult/gastroccult occur with iron, red fruits, rare meat, iodine.
- False negative hemoccult/gastroccult occur with vitamin C, antacids, bile.

Lower GI Bleeding

Most common source of massive lower GI bleeding is an upper GI site, therefore all patients require NG tube. 80-90% of lower bleeding will stop without therapy.

Diverticulosis - 75% of bleeds are from right colon. Bleeding is arterial, and often massive. Pain is mild and crampy in nature. 50% rebleed & 20% require surgery.

Angiodysplasia - Acquired disorder of unknown cause. Lesions are usually in cecum and ascending colon. Barium studies and colonoscopy may not show these lesions. Selective mesenteric angiography is accurate.

Most Common Sources of Lower GI Bleeding[1]	
Diverticulosis	35%
Angiodysplasia	30%
Cancer polyps	10%
Rectal disease	7%
Other causes	3%
Undiagnosed	15%
[1]excluding upper GI	

Assessment and Management of Lower GI Bleeding

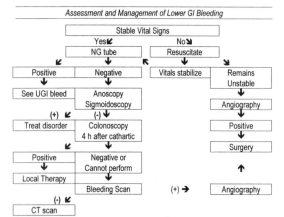

Anemia

Anemia Differential Diagnosis

Microcytic (MCV < 81)[1]	Normocytic (MCV 81-100)[1]	Macrocytic (MCV > 100)[1]
• Low iron RDW[2] > 14% • Thalassemia RDW < 14% • Chronic inflammation • Sideroblastic anemia • Lead poisoning • B6 deficiency		• Folate/B12 deficiency • Liver disease • Hypothyroidism

	High reticulocyte count[3]	Normal or ↓ reticulocytes
	• Subacute or chronic blood loss • Autoimmune hemolysis • Cardiac valves • DIC or HUS[4] • Enzyme deficient(G6PD) • Spherocytosis • Hemoglobinopathy (e.g. sickle cell disease)	• Acute blood loss • Chronic disease • Renal Insufficiency • Bone marrow suppression (e.g. medications, viral, or cancer)

[1] MCV – mean corpuscular volume in μm[3]
[2] RDW – red blood cell distribution width
[3] reticulocyte count X (Hct measured/Normal Hct)
[4] DIC – disseminated intravascular coagulation, HUS – hemolytic uremic syndrome

---

Sickle Cell Anemia

Diagnostic Studies in Sickle Cell Disease

- A routine Hb is recommended in most to assess severity or change of anemia.
- A white blood cell count often will be elevated due to sickle crisis alone.
- Evaluate for precipitant for crisis (e.g., infection, or dehydration).
- Consider a reticulocyte count if aplastic crisis suspected (Mean reticulocyte count for sickle cell patient is 12%, in aplastic crises it may be <3-5%).
- Urine specific gravity is not a useful test for dehydration, as it may be low from isosthenuria (inability to concentrate urine).

Admission Criteria for Sickle Cell Disease

- Acute chest syndrome – chest pain with pulmonary infiltrate from either infection or pulmonary infarct
- Aplastic crisis
- Serious bacterial infection
- Stroke
- Priapism
- Unable to take fluids orally or inadequate pain control in the ED
- Patients with uncertain diagnoses

Management of Sickle (SS) Cell Complications

Abdominal pain	• Patients with SS have ↑ risk for developing cholecystitis, mesenteric ischemia, or a perforated viscus. Splenic sequestration is rare in adults. Consider CT, ultrasound and surgical consultation (esp. if pain not typical of normal crisis).
Aplastic crisis	• Exclude reversible cause (medications) and transfuse for severe anemia (Hb < 6-7 g/dl) or cardiopulmonary distress.
Pain crisis	• Administer O_2 at 2-4 Liters. • IV ½NS at 150-200 ml/h (if mild pain, ± PO hydration) • IV narcotics titrated to pain relief (PO narcotics if mild pain)
Priapism	• Treat as pain crisis above. • Exchange transfusion to keep Hb S < 30% before surgery
Acute chest syndrome	• Admit all patients with a pulmonary infiltrate to the hospital. • Chest syndrome is a pulmonary infarct due to vaso-occlusion that may become infected. • Treat as pain crisis with IV antibiotics. Do not anti-coagulate. • Avoid angiography, as this procedures worsens sickling
Sepsis	• Admit all patients with invasive bacterial infections.
Sickle cell stroke	• Obtain CT ± spinal tap, Administer IV NS. • Exchange transfusion – keep HbS <30% total blood volume

---

Bleeding Disorders

Platelet and *capillary* disorders cause mucous membrane bleeds (GI, epistaxis, prolonged bleed with cuts, petechiae (↑BT and abnormal platelets). *Coagulation* disorders cause hemorrhage of deep muscle, CNS, hemarthrosis, and ↑PT/PTT.

Factor VIII and IX Deficiency (Hemophilia A and B)
Severity of Bleeding and Dose of Factor VIII and IX

Severity	Specific Injury	Desired activity	Dose Factor 8	Dose Factor 9
Severe	CNS, GI bleed, major trauma, retroperitoneal or retropharyngeal bleed, pending surgery	80-100%	40-50 Units/kg	80-100 Units/kg
Moderate	Mild head trauma, deep muscle bleed, hip or groin injury, mouth or dental bleed, hematuria	40-50%	20-25 Units/kg	40-50 Units/kg
Mild	Laceration, common joint bleed, tissue or muscle bleed	20-40%	10-20 Units/kg	20-40 Units/kg

Replacement Factors and Medications used for Hemophilia

Medication	Dose
amino-caproic acid (*Amicar*)	• Use - to prepare for dental procedures • 100 mg/kg PO q 6 hours for 6 days • Alternately, use cyclokapron 25 mg/kg PO x 6 days
DDAVP *Desmopressin*	• 0.3 µg/kg in 50 ml NS IV over 30 minutes • Possibly effective via nasal spray or SC injection, recommended only if baseline activity > 10%
Factor VIII	• [desired activity level (%) – baseline activity level (%)] ÷2 • 1 unit/kg factor 8 will↑activity level 2% (T½ = 12 hours)[1]
Factor IX	• desired activity level (%) - baseline activity level (%) • 1 unit/kg factor 9 will↑activity level 1% (T½ = 24 hours) [1]
prednisone	• 2 mg/kg/day PO x 2 days is useful if mild hematuria

[1] T½ = half life and dosing frequency

Causes of Abnormal Bleeding Tests [1]

Lab Value	Causes
thrombocytopenia ↓ platelet count (<150,000/ml)	Heparin, ↓ platelet production, splenic sequestration, platelet destruction (drugs, collagen vascular disease, , ITP, DIC, TTP, HUS)
platelet dysfunction (with normal count)	Adhesion defects (e.g. von Willibrand's disease) or aggregation defects (e.g. thrombasthenia), renal failure
↑ BT (>9 minutes)	All platelet disorders, DIC, ITP, uremia, liver failure, aspirin
↑ PTT (>35 sec)	Coagulation pathway defects (common factors 2, 5, 10, intrinsic 8, 9, 11, 12), DIC, liver failure, heparin
↑ PT (>12-13 sec)	Coagulation pathway defects (common factors 2, 5, 10, extrinsic 7) DIC, liver failure, *Coumadin*
↑ TT (>8-10 sec)	DIC, liver failure or uremia, heparin
↓ fibrinogen, ↑ FSP	ITP, liver failure

[1] BT-bleeding time, TT-Thrombin time, PTT-partial thromboplastin time, PT-prothrombin time, DIC-disseminated intravascular coagulopathy, ITP-idiopathic thrombocytopenic purpura, TTP-thrombotic thrombocytopenic purpura, HUS-hemolytic uremic syndrome.

BLOOD PRODUCTS

	Cryoprecipitate
Features	• 1 bag(10 ml) has 50-100 units of factor 8 activity. There are 10 donors/bag. It has fibrinogen, von Willibrand's factor, factor 8 + 13.
Indications	• Hypofibrinogenemia if fibrinogen < 100 mg/dl. • Von Willebrand's (vW) disease & active bleeding - if DDAVP is unavailable or factor 8 concentrate with vW factor is unavailable. • Hemophilia A + unavailable monoclonal or viral inactivated factor 8 • Fibronectin replacement for healing in trauma, burns, or sepsis
Dose	• 2-4 bags for every 10 kg of bodyweight or 10-20 bags at a time

	Fresh frozen plasma (FFP)
Features	• Contains all coagulation factors. 40 ml/kg raises activity of any factor to 100%. This may cause fluid overload. ABO compatibility is mandatory although cross matching prior to transfusion is not.
Indications	• Coagulation protein deficiency if factor concentrates unavailable • Reversal of *Coumadin* toxicity or active bleed with liver disease • Bleeding and coagulopathy with unknown cause
Dose	• If bleeding from vitamin K deficiency (liver disease) administer 10-25 ml/kg. 10-15 ml/kg will raise factor 8 levels 15-20%.

	Packed Red Blood Cells (PRBC's)
Features	• Fewer antigens are present in PRBC's compared to whole blood. • *Leukocyte poor* – use if transplant recipient or candidate, or 2 febrile non-hemolytic reaction • *Washed* – use if prior anaphylaxis due to IgA or other proteins. • *Frozen deglycerolized* - purest RBC product, use if reaction to washed RBC's or a transfusion reaction from Anti-IgA antibodies
Indications	• Acute hemorrhage or chronic anemia with hemoglobin < 7 g/dl • Symptomatic or underlying cardiopulmonary disease + Hb < 7 g/dl
Dose	• One unit raises hemoglobin by 1g/dl or hematocrit by 3%. • ≥ 2 units are needed in most circumstances.

	Platelet concentrate
Features	• 1 unit (pack) = 5-10,000 platelets. Platelets are not refrigerated & survive 7 days. ABO cross-match is not necessary, but preferred.
Indications	• Level < 10,000/μL unless antiplatelet antibodies • Level < 50,000/μL if major surgery, significant bleed, major trauma • Level - 10,000-50,000/μL if concurrent liver or renal disease that is causing platelet dysfunction
Dose	• 6 platelet packs (250-300 ml) or one plateletpheresis pack should raise platelet count by 50,000-60,000/uL.

BLOOD PRODUCTS continued

Whole blood	
Features	• Has no WBC's and only 20% platelets after 24h. Factors 5 and 8 ↓60% and RBC's↓ 30% after 21 days. With storage, K+ and NH₄ ↑ (beware in liver failure) and Ca⁺²↓.
Indications	• Massive exsanguination, although this is better treated with PRBC's/crystalloid with replacement of specific components prn
Dose	• One unit contains 450-500 ml of whole blood

Transfusion Reactions
Crossmatching and ordering blood products:
- Type-specific non-crossmatched blood causes fatality in 1 in 30 million transfusions (most commonly due to labeling or patient identification error).
- Non-ABO antibodies occur in 0.04% of non-transfused and 0.3% of previously transfused.

Hemolytic transfusion reactions
- Occur in 1/40,000 transfusions and are usually due to ABO incompatibility.
- *Clinical Features* - palpitations, abdominal and back pain, syncope, and a sensation of doom. Consider in those with a temperature rise of ≥ 2C.
- *Management* - Immediately stop transfusion, and look for hemoglobinemia and hemoglobinuria. Perform direct antiglobulin (Coomb's test), haptoglobin, peripheral smear, serum bilirubin, and repeat antibody screen and crossmatch. Keep urine output at 100 ml/hour and consider alkalization of the urine to limit acute renal failure. Mannitol is not helpful, as it increases urine flow by decreasing tubular reabsorption without improving renal perfusion.

Anaphylactic reaction
- Almost exclusively occurs in those with Anti-IgA antibodies (1/70 people).
- *Clinical Features* - It usually begins after the first few ml of blood with afebrile flushing, wheezing, cramps, vomiting, diarrhea, and hypotension.
- *Management* - stop transfusion and treat with *Benadryl*, epinephrine & steroids.

Febrile non-hemolytic reactions
- *Clinical Features* - occurs during or soon after starting 3-4% of transfusions, most common if multiply transfused or multiparous with anti-leukocyte antibodies.
- *Management* - Stop transfusion and treat as transfusion reaction.

Urticarial reactions
- *Clinical Features* - causes local erythema, hives and itching.
- *Management* - Further evaluation unnecessary unless fever, chills, or other adverse effects are present. This is the only type of transfusion reaction in which the infusion can continue.

Hyperviscosity Syndrome

Etiology	Diagnosis
↑serum proteins with sludging & ↓ circulation. Common causes: macroglob-ulinemia, myeloma and CML.	• WBC (esp. blasts)>100,000 cells/mm^3 • ↑serum viscosity -Ostwald viscometer • Serum protein electrophoresis
Clinical Features	Management
• Fatigue, headache, somnolence • ↓vision, seizure, deafness, MI, CHF • Retinal bleed and exudates	• IV NS • 2 unit phlebotomy with NS, and packed red blood cell replacement

Spinal Cord Compression

Most often due to lymphoma, lung, breast or prostate cancer. 68% are thoracic, 19% lumbosacral, and 15% cervical spine.

Clinical Features		Diagnosis
Back pain	95%	• Plain films are abnormal in 60-90%
Weakness (usually symmetric)	75%	• MRI or CT or myelography
Autonomic or sensory symptoms	50%	Management[1]
Inability to walk	50%	• Dexamethasone 25 mg IV q 6 hours
Flaccidity, hyporeflexia (early) or	-	• Radiation therapy
spasticity, hyperreflexia (late)	-	• Surgery may be needed for epidural
Bowel/bladder incontinence	-	abscess/bleed, or disc herniation

[1] Steroid and radiation may be indicated if cancer is cause of compression.

Superior Vena Cava Syndrome

Occurs in 3-8% with lung cancer & lymphoma. Symptoms are due to venous hypertension in areas drained by superior vena cava. Death occurs from cerebral edema, airway compromise, or cardiac compromise.

Clinical Features		Diagnosis
Thoracic or neck vein distention	65%	• CXR shows mediastinal mass or parenchymal lung mass in 10%
Shortness of breath	50%	
Tachypnea	40%	• CT is diagnostic
Upper trunk or extremity edema	40%	Management
Cough/dysphagia/chest pain	20%	• Furosemide 40 mg IV
Periorbital or facial edema	-	• Methylprednisolone 1-2 mg/kg mg IV
Stoke's sign (tight shirt collar)	-	• Mediastinal radiation

Tumor Lysis Syndrome

Occurs within 1-2 days of starting chemotherapy or radiation for rapidly growing tumors (esp. leukemias and lymphomas).
Clinical features are due to hyperuricemia (renal failure), ↑K$^+$ (arrhythmias), ↑phosphate (renal failure), and ↓Ca^{+2} (cramping, tetany, confusion, seizures).

Management	Criteria for Hemodialysis
• Hydration with NS • Allopurinol 10-200 mg PO/day • Alkalinize serum with NaHCO$_3$ to urine pH ≥ 7.0 • Dialysis	• K$^+$ > 6 mEq/L • Creatinine > 10 mg/dl • Uric acid > 10 mg/dl • Symptomatic hypocalcemia • Serum phosphorus > 10 mg/dl

Hypertensive Emergencies

Hypertensive emergency - an elevated BP with end-organ damage or dysfunction. Treatment goal is to reduce MAP by 20-25% % in 30-60 min.

Hypertensive urgency - an elevated BP to level that may potentially be harmful if sustained (usually diastolic BP > 115 mm Hg) without end-organ damage. Treatment goal is to reduce pressure gradually within 24-48 h to normal for patient.

<u>Mean Arterial Pressure (MAP)</u> – diastolic BP (DBP) + 1/3 pulse pressure (SBP-DBP)

Hypertensive Emergencies

- *Catecholamine-induced hypertension* - Acute ↑catecholamines with acute sympathetic overactivity and hypertension due to pheochromocytomas, monoamine oxidase inhibitors, sympathomimetics, clonidine or β blocker withdrawal. Treat with labetolol or α-blockers (e.g. phentolamine).
- *Left ventricular failure and coronary insufficiency* - ↑ afterload can lead to pulmonary edema, and myocardial ischemia by increasing O_2 demand and ↓ coronary flow. Nitroglycerin IV is the drug of choice. See page 16 for further recommendations regarding treatment of acute pulmonary edema.
- *Hypertensive Encephalopathy* - headache, vomiting, & altered mental status due to cerebral hyperperfusion with loss of the blood brain barrier and ability to autoregulate cerebral blood flow. Late findings: general cerebral vasodilation, ↓blood flow, cerebral edema, papilledema, or exudates. Treat with sodium nitroprusside (*Nipride*) or labetolol (*Normodyne*). Lower MAP so cerebral blood flow normalizes within 30-60 min. Do not lower MAP to < 120 mm Hg.
- *Pregnancy-induced Hypertension* - see page 68.
- *Renal failure* - ↓ renal function due to ↑ BP is a hypertensive emergency. Proteinuria, red cells, red cell casts and ↑ BUN/creatinine occur.
- *Thoracic dissection* – Treat with labetolol or (sodium nitroprusside + esmolol).

Oral Agents For Use in Hypertensive Urgencies

- Debate exists as to whether any acute treatment is needed in the ED setting.
- <u>captopril</u> (*Capoten*) - 25 mg PO bid/tid (after 6.25 mg test dose). Onset is 30 min, peak effect 1-1.5 hours and duration 4-6 hours.
- <u>clonidine</u> (*Catapres*) - 0.2 mg PO. Repeat 0.1 mg PO q 1-2 h until diastolic BP is < 115 mmHg or maximum of 0.7 mg administered. Onset is 30-60 min, peak effect 2-4 hours and duration 6-8 hours. It is NOT necessary to initiate therapy with clonidine after its use in the ED.
- <u>nifedipine</u> (*Procardia*) - can precipitously ↓ BP causing MI, or stroke. Do not use sublingual route in the Emergency Department.
- <u>labetolol</u> (*Normodyne*) – 100-200 mg PO. Onset is 15-30 min, peak is 1-3 hours, and duration is 8-12 hours. *Emerg Med Clin North Am* 1995; 13:973.

Drugs in Hypertensive Emergencies

Drug	Dose and route	Mechanism	Onset	Duration	Features
enalaprilat (Vasotec)	1.25-5 mg IV over 5 min, administered q 6 hours	ACE inhibitor	15 min	6 hours	Avoid in renal artery stenosis, useful if ↑ renin (scleroderma)
esmolol (Brevibloc)	500 µg/kg IV over 1st min, then titrate 50-200 µg/kg/min	β-blockade	seconds	half-life = 9 min	Worsens bronchospasm, heart blocks, & congestive heart failure
fenoldopam (Corlopam)	0.1-2.0 µg/min IV	Dopamine-1 receptor agonist	4 min	10 min	↑ renal flow, & Na⁺ excretion, esp. useful if ↓ renal function
hydralazine (Apresoline)	5-10 mg IV q 30-60 min or 10-50 mg IM	Arteriolar dilator	<30 min	4-12h	Causes tachycardia, headache
labetalol (Normodyne)	Start at 0.25 mg/kg IV and double dose q15min prn to maximum of 2.0 mg/kg	α and β blockade in 1:7 ratio	seconds	4-8h	Worsens bronchospasm, heart blocks, & congestive heart failure
nicardipine (Cardene)	Start at 2-4 mg/h IV, ↑1-2 mg/h q 15 min. Max 15mg/h	Calcium channel blocker	1-5 min	20 min	Rarely precipitates angina, ↑HR and ↑ICP
nitroglycerin (Tridil)	5-200 µg/min	Direct vasodilator	2-5 min	5-10 min	May ↑heart rate, and ↓BP
propranolol (Inderal)	1 mg IV over 1 min q 5 min up to maximum of 5-8 mg	β-blockade	seconds	up to 8h	Worsens bronchospasm, heart blocks, & congestive heart failure
phentolamine (Regitine)	2-10 mg IV, repeat q 5-15 min	α-blocker	1-2 min	30-60 min	tachycardia in pheochromocytoma
sodium nitroprusside (Nipride)	0.5-8 µg/kg/min infusion	Arterial and venous dilator	seconds	1-3 min	no ↓cardiac output, possible cyanide toxicity and ↑ICP

sec=seconds, min=minutes, h=hours, mo=months, mg=milligrams, µg=micrograms, IV=intravenous, PO=oral, SL=sublingual, IM=intramuscular

Occupational Exposure to Human Immunodeficiency Virus (HIV)

- Highest risk for transmission of HIV: (1) scalpel or needle visibly contaminated with patient's blood, (2) needle placed directly in vein or artery, (3) deep puncture or wound to health care worker (4) terminal illness in source patient.
- ZDV reduces transmission by ~ 79%. Begin prophylaxis ≤ 2-8 h from exposure.

Provisional Public Health Service Recommendations for Chemoprophylaxis after Occupational Exposure to HIV. (CDC. MMWR. 1996; 45(22): 468)

Exposure	Source Material	Prophylaxis?	Drug Regimen [1]
Percutaneous *HIV risk* ~ 0.3%	Blood		
	Highest risk[2]	Recommend	ZDV + 3TC + IDV
	Increased risk[2]	Recommend	ZDV + 3TC ± IDV
	No increased risk[2]	Offer	ZDV + 3TC
	Fluid has visible blood or other infectious fluid[3]	Offer	ZDV + 3TC
	Other fluid (e.g. urine)	Do not offer	
Mucous membrane *HIV risk* ~ 0.1%	Blood	Offer	ZDV + 3TC ± IDV
	Fluid has visible blood or other infectious fluid[3]	Offer	ZDV ± 3TC
	Other fluid (e.g. urine)	Do not offer	
Skin with ↑ risk[4] *HIV risk* < 0.1%	Blood	Offer	ZDV + 3TC ± IDV
	Fluid has visible blood or other infectious fluid	Offer	ZDV ± 3TC
	Other fluid (e.g. urine)	Do not offer	

1 ZDV – zidovudine, 3TC – lamivudine, IDV - indinavir

2 <u>Highest risk</u> – ↑blood volume (e.g. deep injury with ↑diameter hollow needle) AND blood with ↑ titer HIV (e.g. source patient is end-stage, or has↑viral load)
<u>Increased risk</u> - Exposure to ↑blood volume or blood with ↑HIV titer
<u>No increased risk</u> - Neither exposure to large blood volume or high HIV titer

3 Semen, vaginal secretions, CSF, synovial, pleural, peritoneal, pericardial, amniotic fluid

4 Increased risk (for skin) = exposures with high HIV titer, prolonged contact, extensive area, or area in which skin integrity is visibly compromised.

Protocol and Drug Dosing for HIV Exposure

◆ Draw HIV, CBC, liver+renal function, βhCG ± hepatitis exposure work up (pg 52)	
◆ Repeat CBC, liver + renal tests at 2 weeks, and HIV at 6 and 12 weeks, + 12 mo.	
zidovudine(ZDV)	200 mg PO TID X 4 weeks
lamivudine(3TC)	150 mg PO BID X 4 weeks
indinavir (IDV)	800 mg POTID X 4 weeks (may substitute saquinavir 600 mg PO tid)

Most common short term side effects: *ZDV* - GI, fatigue, headache; *3TC* - GI, pancreatitis, *IDV* - GI, high bilirubin, and kidney stones (may be limited by drinking ≥ 1.5 L H$_2$O/day).

Hepatitis B Exposure

Type of exposure	Status of source is	Treatment if exposed patient is	
		Unvaccinated	Vaccinated
percutaneous or mucosal	HBsAg +	HBIG, HBV	HBV & HBIG if exposed HBsAb -
known source	high risk for HBsAg +	HBV and HBIG if source HBsAg +	HBV & HBIG if source HBsAg+ & exposed HBsAb-
known source	low risk for HBsAg +	HBV	none
unknown	unknown	HBV	none
sex / perinatal	HBsAg +	HBIG, HBV	none
house/work	HBsAg +	none	none

HBIG = hepatitis B immune globulin. Dose 0.06 ml/kg IM
HBV = hepatitis B vaccine. Dose : 1 ml IM in deltoid initially, repeat in 1 & 6 mo.
<u>Hepatitis C exposure</u>: Administer immune serum globulin (ISG) 0.06 ml/kg IM.
<u>Hepatitis A exposure</u>: Administer ISG 0.02 ml/kg IM for exposure through close personal contact, employee at day care center, or contaminated food within 2 wks.

Tetanus Immunization

Previous tetanus immunizations	Tetanus prone wound	Non tetanus prone wound
Uncertain or <3	dT, TIG[1]	dT
3 or more	dT if >5y since last dose	dT if >10y since last dose

[1]Tetanus immune globulin. Dose of TIG – 250 units IM at site other than for dT.

Postexposure Rabies Prophylaxis

Rabies prophylaxis only indicated if there is a bite or other salivary exposure from a carnivore or bat. No prophylaxis is needed if the exposure is nonsalivary or if the animal is a bird, reptile, or rodent.

- HDCV (human diploid cell vaccine) dose - 1 ml IM, administered on days 0, 3, 7, 14, & 28. Administer vaccine in deltoid, not buttock.
- RIG (rabies immune globulin) dose - 20 International units/kg with ½ infiltrated SC around the wound and the remainder in the gluteus IM. Do not give near the site of the 1st HDCV injection.

		Is animal a dog or cat?	
		YES	NO, other
Was Animal captured?	NO, escaped	Give RIG & HDCV only if rabies risk for given species in locale.	Treat with RIG and full course of HDCV.
	YES, captured	Observe animal for 10 days. If abnormal behavior, sacrifice and treat patient with RIG & HDCV. Discontinue treatment if animal pathology negative for rabies.	Sacrifice animal and begin RIG and HDCV. Discontinue treatment if pathology negative for rabies.

ADULT Antibiotic Therapy for Sepsis Based on Suspected Organ System (See page 54-56 for DOSING)

Source	Usual Pathogens	Initial Antibiotics	If Penicillin Allergic
Abdomen			
Biliary tract Pelvis Ileum/colon	E. coli, Klebsiella, enterococci Bacteroides fragilis	anti-pseudomonal penicillin (piperacillin, mezlocillin, ticarcillin) or cefoperazone, or PBLI[1]	(metronidazole or clindamycin) + (aminoglycoside or Aztreonam or quinolone or cefipime)
Liver	E. coli,, Bacteroides fragilis	(metronidazole or clindamycin) + (aminoglycoside or aztreonam or quinolone or cefipime or PBLI[1])	(metronidazole or clindamycin) + (aminoglycoside or aztreonam or quinolone)
Genitourinary			
Bladder/kidneys	E. coli, enterococcus, Pseudomonas	ampicillin + (aminoglycoside or anti-pseudomonal penicillin or PBLI[1])	vancomycin + (aminoglycoside or aztreonam)
Prostate	E. coli, enterococcus (gram + organism requires ampicillin)	trimethoprim/sulfamethoxazole or quinolone or PBLI[1]	quinolone or doxycycline trimethoprim/sulfamethoxazole
Urologic instruments	E. coli, P. aueroginosa	PBLI[1] or quinolone or aminoglycoside or aztreonam	quinolone or AG or aztreonam
Intravenous (IV) line	S. aureus, S epidermidis, Klebsiella, Enterobacter, Serratia	(cefipime or vancomycin) + (aminoglycoside or aztreonam or quinolone)	(imipenem or vancomycin) + (aminoglycoside or aztreonam or quinolone)
IV grafts or shunts	S. aureus	nafcillin or clindamycin	clindamycin or vancomycin or teicoplanin
Meningitis or Pneumonia		See page 55,56	See page 55,56

[1]PBLI - penicillin-beta-lactamase inhibitor (e.g. piperacillin/tazobactam, ticarcillin/clavulanate, or ampicillin/sulbactam)

Antimicrobial Therapy for Specific Infections in Adults[1]

Infection	Treatment
Bite infection – dog or cat	• *Augmentin* 875 mg PO bid x 10 days **OR** penicillin 250 mg qid + dicloxacillin 250 mg PO qid **OR** doxycycline 100 mg PO bid X 10 days
Bite infection - human	• Oral - *Augmentin* 875 mg PO bid x 5d (prophylaxis) • IV - *Unasyn* 1.5-3 g IV q6h **OR** cefoxitin 1-2 g IV q8h • If *Eikinella* - *Cleocin* 600-900 mg IV q8h **AND** IV FQ[2]
Cat scratch disease	• *Septra* DS 1 PO bid x 14 days **OR** rifampin 10 mg/kg PO bid-tid X 14 days
Cellulitis – uncomplicated healthy patient	• Oral - dicloxacillin 250-500 mg PO qid x 10d **OR** cephalexin 250-500 mg PO qid x 10d **OR** macrolide[3] • IV - nafcillin 2 g IV q 4 h **OR** *Ancef* 1 g IV q8h
Cellulitis – diabetic, alcohol	• Oral – *Augmentin* 875 mg PO bid **OR** IV/IM 3rd Cp[4] • IV – *Primaxin* 0.5-1 g IV q 6-8 h **OR** *Trovan* IV
Cellulitis – lake/sea H₂0	• Oral: *Septra* 1 DS PO bid x 10 days **OR** FQ[2] x 10 days • IV – aminoglycoside [see page 58]
Chancroid	• azithromycin 1g PO **OR** ceftriaxone 250 mg IM
Chlamydia - urethritis or simple cervicitis	• azithromycin 1 g PO **OR** doxycycline 100 mg PO bid x 7-10 days **OR** erythromycin 500 mg PO qid x 7-10d **OR** tetracycline 500 mg PO qid x 7-10 d **OR** *Trovan* 200 mg PO q day x 5 days
Dental infection	• *Augmentin* 875 mg PO bid **OR** *Cleocin* 300 mg PO qid **OR** penicillin (↑resistance) 250-500 mg PO qid **OR** erythromycin 250-500 mg PO qid x 10 days
Diverticulitis – outpatient	• *Septra* DS 1 PO bid **OR** *Cipro* 500 mg PO bid • **AND** metronidazole 500 mg PO qid at least 7-10 days
Diverticulitis – inpatient	• (cefoxitin 1-2 g IV q6-8h **OR** anti-pseudomonal aminoglycoside [pg 58]) **AND** *Cleocin* 600-900 mg IV q8h
Epididymitis – all ages	• *Cipro* 500 mg PO bid **OR** *Floxin* 300 mg PO bid **OR** *Trovan* 200 mg PO qd x 10-14 days
Epididymitis ≤ 35 years	• see PID – outpatient treatment
Gangrene – Gas, Fournier's, or Necrotizing fasciitis[5]	• *Cleocin* 900 mg IV q8h **AND** penicillin G 4 million units IV q 4-6 hours • **OR** *Unasyn* 3 g IV q 6h **OR** *Timentin* 3.1 g IV q 4-6 hours **OR** *Primaxin* 0.5-1 g IV q6-8h

Infection	Treatment
Gonorrhea – *excluding invasive disease (excluding PID, arthritis etc.)*	• <u>One dose PO of any of the following</u>: azithromycin 2 g, cefixime 400 mg, *Cipro* 500 mg, *Raxar* 400 mg, *Floxin* 400 mg, *Trovan*100 mg • **OR** ceftriaxone 250 mg IM
Herpes – simplex *treat for half of <u>primary</u> time period recurrent simplex*	• <u>Primary</u> - acyclovir (*Zovirax*) 400 mg PO tid x 10 days **OR** valacyclovir (*Valtrex*) 1 g PO bid x 10 days • <u>Prophylaxis</u> - acyclovir 400 mg PO bid **OR** famciclovir 250 mg PO bid **OR** valacyclovir 500 mg PO qd
Herpes – zoster *if immunocompromised or ill consider IV therapy*	• acyclovir 800 mg PO 5 x per day x 7-10 days **OR** famciclovir 500 mg PO tid x 7 days **OR** valacyclovir 1 g PO tid x 7 days
Influenza A *start therapy within 48h of symptoms*	• amantidine (A) **OR** rimantidine (R) 100 mg PO bid x 5d • > 65 years: A 100 mg PO qd **OR** R 100-200 mg PO/day
Lymphogranuloma venerum (LGV)	• doxycycline 100 mg PO bid x 21 days **OR** erythromycin 500 mg PO qid x 21 days
Mastitis	• <u>Oral</u> - dicloxacillin **OR** cephalexin 250-500 mg PO qid • <u>IV</u> - cefazolin 1 g IV q6h
Meningitis - bacterial *< 50 years and healthy*	• cefotaxime 2 g IV q4-6h **OR** ceftriaxone 2 g IV q12h • **AND** vancomycin 1g IV q12h ± steroids (*controversial*)
Meningitis – bacterial *> 50 years or unhealthy*	• ceftriaxone 2 g IV q12h **OR** cefotaxime 2 g IV q4-6h • **AND** ampicillin 2 g IV q4h ± steroids (*controversial*)
Neutropenic fever	• anti-pseudomonal aminoglycoside [page 58] **AND** (piperacillin 3-4 g IV q4-6h **OR** ticarcillin 3 g IV q 4-6h) **OR** *Fortaz* 1-2 g IV q4-6h **OR** *Primaxin* 0.5-1 g IV q6h • **ADD** vancomycin 1g IV q12h if central or peripheral line
Osteomyelitis - healthy	• nafcillin **OR** oxacillin 2g IV q4h **OR** cefazolin 2g IV q6h
Osteomyelitis – *if IV drug user, or dialysis, or immunocompromised*	• *Unasyn* 1.5-3 g IV q6h **OR** *Timentin* 3.1 g IV q4-8h **OR** *Zosyn* 3.375 g IV q 6-8h • **AND** *Cipro* 200-400 mg IV q12h ± *Vancocin* 1g IV q12h
Otitis media	• amoxicillin 250 mg PO tid x 7-10 d **OR** *Septra* 1 DS PO bid x 7-10 days, **OR** *Augmentin* 500-875 mg PO bid, **OR** macrolide[3]
Peritonitis – *bowel perforation*	• *Cleocin* 600-900 mg IV q8h **OR** metronidazole 1 g IV 1st dose, then 500 mg IV q6h • **AND** 3rd Cp[4] **OR** IV FQ[2] **OR** aminoglycoside [pg 58] **OR** *Pipracil* 3-4 g IV q 4-6h **OR** *Ticar* 3-4 g IV q4-6h • <u>Single agent</u> - *Timentin*, **OR** *Unasyn* **OR** *Zosyn* (see doses under osteomyelitis) **OR** IV FQ[2] **OR** 3rd Cp[4]

Infection	Treatment
Peritonitis - *spontaneous*	• cefotaxime 2 g IV q8h **OR** *Unasyn* 1.5-3 g IV q6h **OR** *Timentin* 3.1 g IV q6h **OR** *Zosyn* 3.375 g IV q 6-8h
Pharyngitis *If group A strep. likely*	• Benzathine penicillin (*Bicillin LA*) 1.2-2.4 million units IM **OR** penicillin VK **OR** cephalexin 250-500 mg PO qid x 10 days **OR** cefadroxil 1g qd x 10 days **OR** macrolide[5]
Pelvic inflammatory disease (PID) – *inpatient treatment*	• (cefoxitin 2g IV q 6 h **OR** cefotetan 2g IV q12h) **AND** doxycycline 100 mg PO or IV q 12h x 14 days • **OR** *Cleocin* 900 mg IV q 8h **AND** gentamicin [page 58]. After discharge, doxycycline 100 mg PO bid ± *Cleocin* 450 mg PO qid x 14 days
PID – *outpatient treatment*	• ceftriaxone 250 IM **AND** (doxycycline 100 mg PO bid x 10-14 d **OR** *Trovan* 200 mg PO qd x 14d) • **OR** *Floxin* 400 mg PO bid x 14 days **AND** (*Cleocin* 450 mg PO qid **OR** metronidazole 500 mg PO bid x 14 days)
Pneumonia – *healthy, < 60 years old (community acquired)*	• macrolide[3] **OR** doxycycline 100 mg PO bid x 10 days **OR** *Levaquin* 500 mg PO qd **OR** *Trovan* 200 mg PO qd **OR** *Raxar* 600 mg **PO** qd x 10 days
Pneumonia – *healthy, > 60, community acquired*	• 3rd Cp[4] **AND** (IV or PO macrolide[3]) • **OR** *Levaquin* IV/PO **OR** *Trovan* IV/PO
Pneumonia – *hospital acquired or very ill*	• (*Timentin* 3.1 g IV q6h **OR** *Zosyn* 3.375 g IV q6-8h) **AND** aminoglycoside [see page 58] • **ADD** macrolide IV **OR** PO if *Legionella* suspected
Pneumonia – *Pneumocystis carinii*	• *Septra* 2 DS PO q8h x 21d (IV dose if ill) **OR** (dapsone 100 mg PO qd **AND** trimethoprim 5 mg/kg PO tid x 21d) • **ADD** prednisone taper for 2-3 weeks. (if pO₂ < 70)
Pneumonia - *Aspiration*	• *Cleocin* 450-900 mg IV q8h **OR** cefoxitin 2 g IV q8h **OR** *Timentin* 3.1 g IV q6h **OR** *Zosyn* 3.375 g IV q6-8h
Prostatitis ≤ 35 years	• see PID - outpatient treatment
Prostatitis > 35 years	• *Septra* 1DS PO bid x 14d **OR** see epididymitis-all ages
Pyelonephritis – *healthy*	• Oral– *Septra* DS 1 PO bid **OR**, *Cipro* 500 mg PO bid, **OR** *Noroxin* 400 mg PO bid, **OR** *Levaquin* 250 mg **OR** *Trovan* 200 mg qd x 14d • IV – (ampicillin 2 g IV q4h **AND** gentamicin [page 58]) **OR** IV FQ[2] **OR** 3rd Cp[4]
Pyelonephritis – *nursing home or Foley catheter*	• ampicillin 2 g IV q4h **AND** gentamicin [page 58] • **OR** IV FQ[2] **OR** *Zosyn* 3.375 g IV q6-8h **OR** *Primaxin* 0.25-1g IV q8h

Infection	Treatment
Sepsis	*See page 53 for suspected source and treatment*
Septic arthritis	• nafcillin **OR** oxacillin 2 g IV q4h • If suspect gonorrhea: 3rd Cp[4]
Sinusitis	• Treat as Otitis Media above
Syphilis – *primary or secondary < 1 year*	• benzathine penicillin *(Bicillin LA)* 2.4 million Units IM **OR** doxycycline 100 mg PO bid x 14d
Syphilis – *secondary >1 year*	• benzathine penicillin *(Bicillin LA)* 2.4 million Units IM q week X 3 **OR** doxycycline 100 mg PO bid x 28 days
Trichomonas	• metronidazole 2 g PO x 1 **OR** 500 mg PO bid x 7 days
Urinary tract infection *Females, non-recurrent*	• Septra 1 DS bid, **OR** Cipro 250 mg bid, **OR** Levaquin 250 mg qd, **OR** Trovan 200 mg qd *(all PO x 3 days)*
Vaginosis, bacterial	• Oral - metronidazole 500 mg PO bid x 7 days **OR** Cleocin 300 mg PO bid x 7 days • Intravaginal - metronidazole gel 2 x per day x 5 days **OR** clindamycin vaginal cream qhs x 5 days
Herpes - varicella	• acyclovir 800 mg PO qid x 5 days (IV therapy if immunocompromised, pneumonia or 3rd trimester)
Vascular infection	• vancomycin 1 g IV q 12 h *(e.g. IV, central line, dialysis)*

1 The decision to use IV or PO regimens is complex. Listed medications are only recommendations. Consult textbooks, recent literature, and experts if uncertain about proper treatment options. Certain diseases (e.g. fasciitis, gangrene, septic arthritis, osteomyelitis) may require surgical treatment. Drug doses may need to be changed or selections altered depending on cultures, renal function, & underlying disease.
2 FQ – fluoroquinolone (e.g. ciprofloxacin, ofloxacin, or trovafloxacin)
3 Macrolides – azithromycin *(Zithromax)* 500 mg PO day1, 250 mg PO days 2-5; clarithromycin *(Biaxin)* 250-500 mg PO bid x 7-10 days, erythromycin 250-500 mg PO qid X 7-10 days.
4 3rd Cp – 3rd generation cephalosporin (e.g. cefotaxime, cefizoxime, ceftriaxone)
5 Gas gangrene, necrotizing fasciitis, Fournier's gangrene, and Meleney's synergistic gangrene require similar antibiotics and surgical debridement. Consider hyperbaric O_2.

Aminoglycoside Dosing with Normal Renal Function[1,2]

amikacin *(Amikin)*	15 mg/kg/d IV divide q8-12h, max dose 1500mg/d.
gentamicin *(Garamycin)*	1 mg/kg IV/IM q8h, or 5mg/kg/d
tobramycin *(Nebcin)*	1 mg/kg IV/IM q 8h.

1 Gentamicin and tobramycin can be given once/day at 5-7 mg/kg IV q 24 h or amikacin can be given at 15 mg/kg q 24h. Administer over 60 min to avoid neuromuscular blockade.

2 Adjust aminoglycoside dosing regimen so peak serum levels (drawn 60 min after start of a 30-60min infusion or 60 min after IM injection)are sufficiently high to be bacter-

Drug	Peak	Trough
amikacin	15-30 µg/ml	< 5-10 µg/ml
gentamicin	6-12 µg/ml	< 2 µg/ml
tobramycin	6-12 µg/ml	< 2 µg/ml

icidal (see *peak*)and below trough levels (drawn 30 min prior to next dose).

Aminoglycoside Dosing in Renal Failure

- **Loading dose** – Administer the same loading dose regardless of renal function.
- *Estimate creatinine clearance* $CL_{cr} = \frac{[140 - age\ (years)] \times weight\ (kg)}{serum\ creatinine\ (mg/dl) \times 72}$
- Multiply above X 0.85 for women
- **Maintenance dose** = Recommended dose above X calculated CL_{cr}/100 ml/min **OR**
- **Maintenance dose** for once daily aminoglycosides, alter 1st maintenance dose timing

Creatinine clearance	Timing of maintenance dose (gentamicin example given)
> 60 ml/min	Normal time for recommended interval (q 24h for gentamicin)
40-59 ml/min	At 1.5 X recommended dosing interval (q 36h for gentamicin)
20-39 ml/min	At 2.0 X recommended dosing interval (q 48h for gentamicin)
Check 12 h level with this regimen. For **subsequent** doses, if 12 h gentamicin or tobramycin level is ≤ 3ug/ml widen the dosing interval to q 24 h, if 3-5 ug/ml administer q 36h if, 5-7 ug/ml administer q 48 h	

Criteria for Diagnosis of Acute Pelvic Inflammatory Disease (PID)

All three of following are necessary for diagnosis plus ≥ 1 below

- History of lower abdominal pain, with lower abdominal tenderness
- Tenderness with motion of the cervix and uterus
- Adnexal tenderness

1 of following is needed for diagnosis (criteria are strict & often miss mild PID cases)

- Temperature > 38 C (100.4 F)
- White blood cell count > 10,000/mm^3 or elevated sedimentation rate
- Purulent material (WBC's or bacteria) on culdocentesis or laparoscopy
- Pelvic abscess or inflammatory complex on bimanual exam or ultrasonography
- Gram stain from endocervix positive for gram negative intracellular diplococci
- > 5 white blood cells per high power field on endocervix gram stain.

Obstet Gynecol 1983; 61: 113.

Differentiation Between Genital Ulcers (see page 54-57 for treatment)

Disease	Ulcer Description	Incubation	Painful	Inguinal Nodes
Syphilis	Indurated, nonclean base, heals on own	≥ 2 weeks	No	Firm, rubbery, tender nodes (painless ulcer)
Herpes simplex	Multiple, small grouped vesicles or ulcers with scalloped borders	2-7 d	Yes	Tender, bilateral lymph nodes
Chancroid	Irregular purulent, undermined edges, no induration, multiple	2-12 days	Yes	Very painful, fluctuant, craters may form, unilocular
Lympho-granuloma venereum	Usually not observed, small and shallow, often heal spontaneously	5-21 days	No	Matted clusters of nodes, unilateral or bi-lateral, multiloculated.

Initial Empiric Antibiotics for Intra-Abdominal Infections

Single agents are recommended if mild-moderate infections:
- Cefoxitin (*Mefoxin*) 1-2g IV, **or** Cefotetan (*Cefotan*) 1-2g IV, **or** Ampicillin sulbactam (*Unasyn*) 1.5-3 g IV, **or** Ticarcillin-clavulanic acid (*Timentin*) 3.1 g IV.

Combinations of antibiotics are recommended for severe infections:
- (1) Antianaerobes (e.g. clindamycin 300-600 mg IV or metronidazole 1 g IV) **PLUS** (2) aminoglycoside (gentamicin 1 mg/kg IV, **or** tobramycin 1 mg/kg IV, **or** amikacin 5 mg/kg IV) **OR**
- (1) Antianaerobe (see above) **PLUS** third generation cephalosporin [e.g. ceftazidime (*Fortaz*) 1-2g IV or ceftriaxone (*Rocephin*) 1-2 g IV].
- **OR** Clindamycin 300-600 mg IV **PLUS** aztreonam (*Azactam*) 1-2 g IV

Surgical Infection Society. *Arch Surg* 1992; 127: 83.

Toxic Shock Syndrome

Toxic shock syndrome is due to toxin (TSST-1) produced by *S. aureus*. TSST-1 sources include tampons (50% of cases), nasal packing, wounds, post partum vaginal colonization and many other sites.

Criteria for Diagnosis - Must have each (•) of following
- Temperature > 38.9 C (102F)
- Systolic BP < 90, orthostatic decrease of Systolic BP 15 mm Hg **or** syncope.
- Rash - diffuse, macular erythroderma, with subsequent desquamation.
- Involvement of *3 of the following* organ systems either clinically **or** by labs.

GI - vomiting, or profuse diarrhea	Muscular - myalgias or ↑ CPK X 2
Renal - ↑ BUN + Cr X 2, sterile pyuria	Heme - platelets < 100,000/mm3
Liver - SGOT, SGPT ↑ X 2	Mucosa - vaginal, conjunctiva, or
CNS - disoriented, nonfocal exam	pharyngeal hyperemia

- Negative serology for Rocky Mountain spotted fever, leptospirosis, measles, hepatitis B, antinuclear antibody, VDRL, monospot, blood, urine, throat cultures.

Management
- Restore intravascular volume with NS. Pressors may need to be added.
- Obtain blood for CBC, platelets, coagulation studies, electrolytes, liver function tests, culture urine, blood ± CSF. Obtain CXR, arterial blood gas, and ECG.
- Search for focus of infection and remove source (e.g. tampon).
- If bleeding, treat coagulopathy with platelets, fresh frozen plasma or transfuse.
- Nafcillin or oxacillin 1-2 g IV q 4 h until clinically improved then oral anti-staphylococcal agents (dicloxacillin, or 1st generation cephalosporin) for 10-14 days. Consider vancomycin if suspect methicillin resistant *S. aureus*. Note: antibiotics only reduce recurrence of toxic shock and do not treat actual disease.

Kidney/Renal Disorders

Studies useful in Determining Etiology of Acute Renal Failure

Test	Pre-renal	Renal	Post-renal
Urine sodium (mEq/L)	< 20	> 40	> 40
Fractional excretion of sodium[1]	< 1%	> 2%	> 2%
Renal failure index[2]	< 1	> 2	> 2
Urine osmolality (mOsm/L)	> 500	< 300	< 400
Urine/serum creatinine ratio	> 40	< 20	< 20
Serum BUN/creatinine ratio	> 20	< 10-20	< 10-20
Renal size by ultrasound	normal	normal	normal or↑
Radionucleide renal scan	↓ uptake ↓ excretion	uptake OK ↓ excretion	uptake OK ↓ excretion

[1] $FE_{Na} = 100$ x (urine Na^+/plasma Na^+) / (urine creatinine/plasma creatinine)
  Normal FE_{Na} is 1-2%

[2] RFI = (urine Na^+) / (urine creatinine / serum creatinine)

Calculation of Creatinine Clearance (CLcr)

- Male CLcr = $\frac{[140 - \text{age (years)}] \times \text{weight (kg)}}{\text{serum creatinine (mg/dl)} \times 72}$
- For women, multiply above result by 0.85.
- Normal creatinine clearance is ~ 100 ml/min

Neurologic Disorders

Acute Weakness (Upper vs. Lower Motor Neuron)

Upper motor neuron (UMN) lesions cause damage to the cortex (e.g. stroke), brain stem, or spinal cord. Lower motor neuron (LMN) lesions damage the anterior horn cells, the neuromuscular junction or muscle (e.g. muscular dystrophies).

	Category	UMN disease	LMN disease
Differentiation of	Muscular deficit	Muscle groups	Individual muscles
upper motor neuron	Reflexes	Increased	Decreased/absent
from lower motor	Tone	Increased	Decreased
neuron disease	Fasciculations	Absent	Present
	Atrophy	Absent/minimal	Present

Assessment of Acute Muscle Weakness

Assess ventilation: FVC should be $\geq$ 15ml/kg and max. inspiratory force > 15cmH$_2$0

Spinal Cord	Peripheral Neuropathy	Myoneural Junction	Muscle disease
Lower limbs weak	Generally weak	Cranial nerves	Generally weak
Absent lower DTR[1]	General areflexia	Generally weak	Weak proximally
Sharp sensory level	Stocking/glove	Fasiculations	Muscles tender
Bladder/bowel	Sensory loss	No sensory loss	No sensory loss
(B/B) incontinence	OK B/B	OK B/B	OK B/B
↓ examples[2]	↓ examples[2]	↓ examples[2]	↓ examples[2]
Transverse myelitis Cord tumor/bleed or abscess or disc herniation	Guillain Barre Porphyria, arsenic toxic neuropathy tick paralysis	Myasthenia gravis Organophosphates Botulism	Polymyositis Alcohol/endocrin myopathy Electrolyte abnl[3]

[1] DTR - deep tendon reflexes, [2] - lists are not comprehensive., [3] - abnormality (K, Na, Ca)

Bell's Palsy

A peripheral 7th cranial nerve palsy. Etiology is usually viral (e.g. herpes), but must exclude Lyme disease, middle ear infection/lesion, CNS mass, or vascular disease.

Clinical Features		Management
Weakness of forehead muscles	100%	• Exclude CNS and otic disease
Maximum deficit in 96 h	>95%	• Prednisone 50 mg PO qd X 5 days
Maximum deficit in 48 h	50%	• Administer *Lacrilube* to eye & patch eye
↑ tearing	68%	shut to prevent corneal abrasion
Mastoid pain	61%	• ± Acyclovir 400 mg PO 5 times/day for
Abnormal taste	57%	10 days (esp. if onset < 3 days)[1]
Hyperacusis	29%	• Follow up with neurologist
↓ tearing	16%	
Numbness (± 5th cranial nerve)	<50%	

[1]*Ann Oto Rhin Laryngol* 1996; 105: 371.

Guillain-Barre

Guillain-Barre is post-infectious autoimmune destruction of peripheral nerves. 85-95% have full recovery (weeks to months after weakness progression stops).

Clinical Features	Diagnosis
• Recent viral illness in 50-67%	• Primarily based on clinical features
• Weakness begins symmetrically in legs and ascends to arms and trunk	• CSF – protein normal or > 400 mg/L
• Weakness onset is rapid	• CSF –white cell count normal or monocytosis
• ↓ or absent deep tendon reflexes	• Nerve conductions study (slowing)
• Face involvement in 25-50%	Management
• Hypesthesias or paresthesias in 33%	• 16-28% require ventilatory support
• Miller-Fischer variant – weakness begins in face and descends with ophthalmoplegia and ataxia	• Plasmaphoresis and/or steroids
	• Watch for embolism (consider SC heparin) and infection

Myasthenia Gravis

An autoimmune disease where antibodies destroy acetylcholine receptor at myoneural junction. Thymus abnormalities (thymoma in 10-25%) are often present.

Clinical Features	
• Ptosis, diplopia, blurring (common)	• Either truncal or extremity weakness
• Dysarthria, dysphagia, jaw muscle weakness, head drooping	• Weakness worsens with repitition
• Asymmetric weakness	• Heat worsens & cold improves weakness (cold pack improves ptosis)
Myasthenic crisis	Crisis Management
• Due to worsening disease with weakness, difficulty swallowing and respiratory insufficiency.	• Tensilon test: edrophonium (*Tensilon*) 1-2 mg IV while on cardiac monitor. If no adverse response, give 8 mg IV. Improvement = myasthenic crisis. Worsening = cholinergic crisis.
• Precipitants – infection, antibiotics Aminoglycosides, tetracycline, clindamycin), CNS depressants, β blockers, quinidine, procainimide, lidocaine, metabolic (↑K,↑Mg, ↓K,↓Ca)	• Assess ventilation – Forced Vital Capacity should be ≥ 15 ml/kg and Maximum inspiratory force should be > 15 cm H_2O
Cholinergic crisis	• Look for and treat precipitants.
• Overdose of anticholinesterase meds.	• Admit all patients with either a myasthenic crisis or with a cholinergic crisis.
• Weakness occurs with SLUDGE (salivation, lacrimation, urination, defecation, GI upset, and emesis)	

Subarachnoid Hemorrhage (SAH)

Saccular (berry) aneurysms are most common cause (> AV malformations, mycotic aneurysms, anticoagulation or vasculitis). *Risks:* family history, pre-eclampsia, atherosclerosis, hypertension, alcohol, cigarettes, aspirin, cocaine. Mean age at rupture is 40-60 years. 56% occur at rest, 25% while working, 10% while sleeping.

Clinical features	
Any headache (H/A)	70%
Warning (sentinel) H/A	55%
Neck pain or stiffness	78%
Altered mental status	53%
3rd cranial nerve deficit	9%
Seizure	3-25%
Focal deficit	19%
No H/A, deficit, or nuchal rigidity	11%

Cooperative Aneurysm Study *Neurology* 1983; 33: 981.

Grade	Hunt and Hess Classification of SAH	Normal CT
I	Asymptomatic, minimal headache (H/A) and mild nuchal rigidity	15%
II	Moderate-severe H/A, nuchal rigidity, cranial nerve deficits only	7%
III	Drowsy, confused or mild focal deficit	4%
IV	Stupor, mild/mod hemiparesis, early decerebrate or vegetative Δ	1%
V	Deep coma, decerebrate rigidity, moribund appearance	0%

SAH Diagnosis	SAH Treatment
• CT abnormal > 95% if onset < 12 h	• Lower ICP (page 110)
• CT abnormal 77% if onset > 12 h	• ↓systolic BP to ≤ 160 mm Hg or
• CSF > 100,000 RBC's/ mm³ (mean)	MAP to ≤ 110 mm Hg
although any # RBC's can be found	• Nimodipine (*Nimotop*) 60 mg PO q4-6
• Xanthochromia (traumatic spinal taps	h to↓vasospasm if *Grade I-III* above
do not cause acute xanthochromia)	• Fosphenytoin/phenytoin prophylaxis
• ECG – peaked, deep or inverted T	• Early angiography & surgical inter-
waves, ↑ QT, or large U waves	vention if *Grade I-III* above

Stroke

Ischemic strokes (85%) are (1) thrombotic (2) embolic or (3) hypoperfusion. Hemorrhagic strokes (15%) are intracerebral or subarachnoid (see below).

Major stroke syndromes

• *Anterior cerebral artery:* paralysis of contralateral leg > arm. Sensory deficits parallel weakness, with altered mentation, gait apraxia, and incontinence.
• *Middle cerebral artery:* paralysis contralateral arm, face > leg. Sensory deficits parallel paralysis, blind (½ visual field), dysphasia, & agnosia.
• *Posterior cerebral artery* (occipital, parietal lobes): Blind in half of visual field, 3rd nerve paralysis, visual agnosia, altered mental status and cortical blindness.
• *Vertebrobasilar artery:* vertigo, nystagmus, dysphagia, facial numbness, dysarthria, contralateral loss of pain, temperature, diplopia, syncope.

Management: (1) Assess breathing, & exclude ↓glucose, ↓O₂. (2) Obtain ECG, CT scan, electrolytes, glucose, and CBC. (3) IV NS if dehydrated unless ↑BP or ICP. (4) Only treat hypertension in ischemic stroke if BP ≥ 220/120. (5) Consider thrombolytics (controversial - see pg 64).

Thrombolytic (rTPA) use in Acute Ischemic Stroke

Indications for rTPA[1] use in Acute Ischemic Stroke[2]	Age 18-80 years
	Onset of symptoms ≤ 3 hours before treatment initiated
	No CT scan evidence of bleeding or major early infarct (below)
	Acute focal neurologic deficits excluding contraindications

[1] rTPA - tissue plasminogen activator. (Streptokinase is NOT used for acute stroke)
[2] Facilities administering rTPA should have ability to manage intracranial bleeding.
Neurology 1996; 47: 835.

Contraindications to rTPA Use in Acute Ischemic Stroke

Any CNS bleed (current or prior history)	CT with major early infarct signs[1]
Recent CNS surgery, trauma, or stroke[2]	Major deficit - NIH stroke scale > 22[a]
Recent myocardial infarction	Rapidly improving neurologic signs
Recent spinal tap, major vessel puncture	Pregnancy or lactating females
Blood glucose < 50 or > 400 mg/dl	*Known bleeding diathesis including:*
Uncontrolled HTN[3] (BP ≥ 185/110)	• *Coumadin* use or PT > 15 (INR >1.7)
Seizure at onset of stroke	• heparin use ≤ 48 hours or high PTT
GI or GU bleeding in prior 21 days	*Isolated mild neurologic deficit (alone)*
Non-CNS surgery in prior 14 days	• ataxia • dysarthria
CNS neoplasm, or aneurysm	• sensory loss • mild weakness

[1] - edema, sulcal effacement, mass effect or possible hemorrhage. [2] - prior 3 months
[3] HTN - hypertension (after treatment), [a] See page 65 for NIH stroke scale.

Protocol for rTPA Administration

- Administer rtPA 0.9 mg/kg (max dose of 90 mg) with 10% given as IV bolus followed by infusion of remaining drug over 60 minutes.
- Monitor arterial blood pressure during ensuing 24 hours

(1) Monitor q 15 min X 1st 2 hours	(3) Then q 60 min for next 16 hours
(2) Then q 30 min for next 6 hours	(4) Treat blood pressure (see below)

- Do not administer aspirin, heparin, *Coumadin*, ticlopidine or other antiplatelet or antithrombotic agents within 24 hours of rtPA treatment.
- Do not place central venous line or perform arterial punctures in first 24 hours.
- Do not place bladder catheter for 30 min or NG tube for 24 hours after infusion.

Management of Hypertension in Patients Receiving Thrombolytics

Systolic BP[1]	Diastolic BP	Treatment - if no contraindications to labetolol use
180-230	105-120	*labetolol* 10 mg IV over 1-2 min. May repeat or double dose q 10-20 min to total dose of 150 mg
> 230	121-140	above dose of *labetolol*. If no response, consider *sodium nitroprusside*[2] (0.5 – 8 µg/kg/min)
	> 140	*sodium nitroprusside*[2] (0.5 – 8 µg/kg/min)

[1] BP - blood pressure in mm Hg taken on two or more readings 5-10 min apart
[2] Check BP q 15 min during use

National Institute of Health Stroke Scale

1a. Level of consciousness (LOC)[1]	Alert	0	8. Plantar reflex	Normal	0
	Drowsy	1		Equivocal	1
	Stuporous	2		Extensor	2
	Coma	3		Bilateral extensor	3
1b. LOC questions *(birthday, today's date?)*	Both correct	0	9. Limb ataxia	Absent	0
	One correct	1		Present in upper or	
	Incorrect	2		Lower	1
1c. LOC commands *(make fist, close eyes)*	Obeys both	0		Present in both	2
	Obeys one	1	10. Sensory	Normal	0
	Incorrect	2		Partial loss	1
2. Pupillary response	Both react	0		Dense loss	2
	One reactive	1	11. Neglect	No neglect	0
	Not reactive	2		Partial neglect	1
3. Best gaze	Normal	0		Complete neglect	2
	Partial palsy	1	12. Dysarthria[2]	Normal articulation	0
	Forced deviation	2		Mild to moderate dysarthria	1
4. Best visual	No loss	0		Near unitelligible or worse	2
	Partial hemianopsia	1	13. Best language	No aphasia	0
	Complete hemianopsia	2		Mild to moderate aphasia	1
5. Facial palsy	None	0		Severe aphasia	2
	Minor	1	14. Change from prior examination		
	Partial	2	Same (S), Better (B), Worse (W)		
	Complete	3	15. Change from baseline		
6. Best motor arm *(Positive drift = if 1 arm pronates or drifts in 10 sec)*	No drift	0	Same (S), Better (B), Worse (W)		
	Drift	1			
	Can't resist gravity	2			
	No effort vs. gravity	3			
7. Best motor Leg	No drift	0			
	Drift	1			
	Can't resist gravity	2			
	No effort vs. gravity	3	*Neurology* 1996; 47: 835.		

1 Drowsy – minor stimulation needed to answer question; lethargic – painful stimuli required; obtunded – totally unresponsive.

2 Dysarthria – slurring from paralysis or incoordination of muscles for speech

3 Aphasia – disturbance in processing language. Patient often uses inappropriate words or nonfluent sentences. Test *receptive aphasia* by having patient follow simple commands and test *expressive aphasia* by identifying objects.

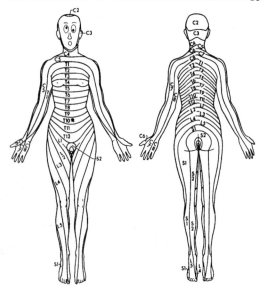

Motor level	Motor function
C1-2	neck flexion
C3	side neck flexion
C4	spontaneous breathing
C5	shoulder abduction/deltoid
C6	biceps, wrist extension
C7	triceps, wrist flexion
C8	thumb ext, ulnar deviation
C8/T1	finger flexion
T1-T12	intercostal and abdominal muscles

Motor level	Motor function
T7-L1	abdominal muscles
T12	cremasteric reflex
L1/L2	hip flexion, psoas
L2/3/4	hip adduction, quads
L4	foot dorsiflexion, foot inversion
L5	great toe dorsiflexion
S1	foot plantar flexion foot eversion
S2-S4	rectal tone

Diagnosis of Ectopic Pregnancy in Clinically Stable Patients

Qualitative βhCG or immediate bedside ultrasound if available
(Immediate laparotomy if in shock and suspect ectopic)

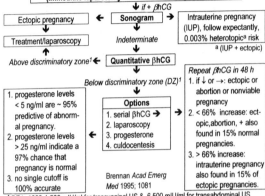

↓ *if + βhCG*

| Ectopic pregnancy | ← | **Sonogram** | → | Intrauterine pregnancy (IUP), follow expectantly, 0.003% heterotopic[a] risk |

↓

Treatment/laparoscopy   *Indeterminate*

↑   ↓

Above discriminatory zone[1] ← **Quantitative βhCG**

Below discriminatory zone (DZ)[1]

↓

1. progesterone levels < 5 ng/ml are ~ 95% predictive of abnormal pregnancy.
2. progesterone levels > 25 ng/ml indicate a 97% chance that pregnancy is normal
3. no single cutoff is 100% accurate

Options
1. serial βhCG →
2. laparoscopy
3. progesterone
4. culdocentesis

Brennan Acad Emerg Med 1995; 1081

Repeat βhCG in 48 h
1. if ↓ or →: ectopic or abortion or nonviable pregnancy
2. < 66% increase: ectopic, abortion, + also found in 15% normal pregnancies.
3. > 66% increase: intrauterine pregnancy also found in 15% of ectopic pregnancies.

[a] (IUP + ectopic)

[1] DZ is 1000-1,500 mIU/ml for transvaginal US & 6,500 mIU/ml for transabdominal US

Ultrasound (US) Findings[1]

Intrauterine pregnancy (IUP)
1. Decidual reaction
2. Gestational sac seen at 4.5 wk with βhCG > 1000-1400 via transvaginal US or 6 wk with βhCG > 6,500 via transabdominal US
3. Yolk sac - see at 5.5 weeks (βhCG > 7200)
4. Fetal pole/heart beat are seen at 5.5 to to 7 weeks (βhCG > 10,800-17,200)

Ectopic pregnancy (% with finding)
1. Empty uterus, decidual reaction, or pseudosac (10-20%)
2. Cul-de-sac fluid (24-63%):echogenic=blood
3. Adnexal mass (60-90%)
4. Echogenic halo around tube (26-68%)
5. Fetal heart activity (8-23%)

Quantitative βhCG in IUP [2,3]

Time	mIU/ml
< 1 week	< 5 - 50
1 - 2 weeks	40 - 300
2 - 3 weeks	100 - 1,000
3 - 4 weeks	500 - 6,000
1 - 2 months	5,000 - 200,000
2 - 3 months	10,000 - 100,000
2nd trimester	3,000 - 50,000
3rd trimester	1,000 - 50,000

[1] Transvaginal sonography unless otherwise stated

[2] Time from conception

[3] Median time for βhCG to turn negative after spontaneous abortion is 16 days (30 days for elective)

Pregnancy Induced Hypertension - Preeclampsia - Eclampsia

Pregnancy induced hypertension (PIH)	
• BP ≥ 140/90 mm Hg **Or** • BP ↑of ≥ 30/15 above prior BP	Measure BP on 2 occasions ≥ 6 hours apart (not practical in the ED)

Pre-eclampsia	Severe pre-eclampsia
• Hypertension with general edema or proteinuria > 20 weeks gestation • Weight gain > 2 lb./week or 6lbs/month is suggestive • Proteinuria occurs late: > 300 mg protein/24h (300 mg/d = 1+ dipstick) or > 1 g/L on 2 urines > 6h apart	• BP > 160/110 mm Hg • Proteinuria ≥ 2+, Cr > 1.2 mg/dl-new • Oliguria (urine output ≤ 500 ml/24h) • Elevated AST/ALT • Platelets < 100,000 cells/uL • Headache, visual Δ, abdominal pain, pulmonary edema, hyperreflexia

HELLP syndrome	ECLAMPSIA
• Hemolytic anemia, Elevated Liver function tests, Low Platelets • Variant of pre-eclampsia with upper abdominal pain and/or vomiting • Hypertension/proteinuria are minimal	• Seizures due to PIH in 3rd trimester or within 3-7 d of delivery (± later) • This is the most common cause of death in Pregnancy Induced Hypertension (PIH)

Treatment of Pre-eclampsia/Eclampsia

• *Seizure prophylaxis* - <u>Load</u> 4-6 g MgSO₄ IV in 100 ml NS over 20 min. <u>Maintenance</u>: Add 20 g MgSO₄ to 500 ml NS and administer at 50 ml/h (2g/h). Continue through labor and 12 h after delivery. <u>Side effects</u>: flushing, headache, blurring, dizziness, ↓reflexes, respiratory and cardiac arrest. Monitor patellar reflexes, respirations and keep urine output ≥ 25 ml/h.
<u>Antidote to MgSO₄ overdose</u>: Calcium gluconate (10%) 10-20 ml slow IV push. <u>Contraindications</u> to MgSO₄: myasthenia gravis, maternal cardiovascular disease, renal impairment, or use of nifedipine, β agonists, and steroids as use of these drugs with MgSO₄ may lead to pulmonary edema/cardiac depression.

• *Seizure treatment* - Barbiturates and benzodiazepines are recommended although both may cause fetal depression. (see page 86).

• *Antihypertensives* - <u>Indications</u> - diastolic BP is ≥ 105 mmHg. <u>Goal</u> - ↓diastolic BP to 90-95 mmHg (lower if baseline diastolic BP is known to be < 75 mmHg).
  1. <u>Hydralazine</u> - 5 mg IV over 1-2 min. Repeat 5-10 mg IV q 20-30 min prn. If a total of 20 mg given without effect, try 2nd drug.
  2. <u>Labetolol</u> - 10 mg IV. Double q 10 min until BP goal or max. 300 mg (total).
  3. <u>Diazoxide</u> - Administer 30 mg IV q 5-15 min prn (max dose 150 mg).

Third Trimester Vaginal Bleeding and Post Partum Hemorrhage

Placental Abruption (Separation of Normal Placenta prior to Birth)

Risk factors	Management
• Hypertension, maternal age > 35 y • Smoking, cocaine use, trauma • Causes 30% of 3rd trimester bleeding	• Avoid digital pelvic examination until placenta previa excluded. • Ultrasound is only 25% sensitive.
Clinical Features	• Administer O_2, and IV NS.
• Vaginal bleeding (dark) 78% • Abdominal pain 66% • Uterine contractions 17% • Fetal death 15% • Maternal DIC[1] -	• Obtain type & crossmatch, PT/PTT, CBC fibrinogen, platelets, fibrin degradation products. • Blood, FFP, platelets prn • Immediate delivery

[1]bedside DIC screen: place 5 ml maternal venous blood in red top tube, DIC if no clots by 6 min

Placenta Previa (20% of 3rd Trimester Bleeding)

Defined	Management
• Implanted placenta over cervical os	• If pre-term – tocolysis with
Clinical Features/Diagnosis	(1) terbutaline 0.25-5 mg SC q2h, or
• Sudden profuse vaginal bleeding	(2) terbutaline 2.5-5 mg PO q2-4h or
• Absence of abdominal pain	(3) ritodrine 10 mg PO q 3-4h or
• Soft non-tender uterus	(4) $MgSO_4$ 4-6 g IV (slow) + 2g/h IV
• **AVOID** digital pelvic examination	• If viable pregnancy (near term) –
• Ultrasound is 95% sensitive	delivery via cesarean section

Postpartum Hemorrhage

Definition	Most common causes
Postpartum hemorrhage is the loss of > 500 ml of blood in 1st 24 h after delivery	• Uterine atony • Cervical and uterine lacerations

Management

1. IV NS, blood prn, oxygen, and fundal massage.
2. oxytocin (*Pitocin*) 10 U IM or 10-40 U in 1L NS at 100-200 ml/h after placental delivery - may ↓BP **or** methylergonovine tartrate (*Methergine*) 0.2 mg IM after placenta delivers - may cause ↑or↓BP, seizures, headaches
3. 15-methyl $PGF_2\alpha$ (*Carboprost*) 0.25 mg IM q 15-90 min to maximum dose of 2 mg. May↓O_2, so apply pulse oximeter. Use caution if ↑BP, cardiac, hepatic, renal, lung disease, epilepsy, ↓Hb or diabetes.
4. Surgery may be needed for severe bleeding.
5. Consider cervical or uterine laceration, uterine rupture, or abnormal placental attachment if continued bleeding.

Rh Isoimmunization

Kleihauer Betke test estimates fetal blood transfused into maternal circulation. (fetal cells/maternal cells X maternal blood volume [L] = fetomaternal hemorrhage [ml]).

(1) <u>RhIG (Rh Immune globulin/RhoGAM)</u> - 1 vial IM is indicated if fetal RBC's possibly entered circulation of Rh negative mother. 1 RhIG vial contains ~ 300 µg of immune globulin and protects against transfusion of 15 ml of Rh^+ packed RBC's. > 1 dose is indicated if > 15 ml of blood is transferred to mom (see Kleihauer Betke).

(2) <u>RhIG (MICRhoGAM, MiniGamulin Rh, HypRho-D Mini Dose)</u> - 1/6 full dose neutralizes 2.5 ml RBC's. Indications - pregnancy termination, or ectopic ≤12weeks.

Indications for RhIG therapy

Rh negative mother and one of the following	
• Delivery of Rh positive infant	• Threatened abortion (*controversial*)
• Abortion or ectopic pregnancy	• Following amniocentesis, chorionic
• Following trauma (even if minor)	villi or umbilical blood sampling
• Any transfusion of Rh positive blood	• At 28 weeks

Emerg Med Clin N Am 1994; 12: 257

Selected Drugs That Can Be Used Safely During Pregnancy
SEE TARASCON Pocket Pharmacopiea for further detail

Condition	Drugs of Choice and Alternative Drugs[2]
Allergic Rhinitis	*Topical:* glucocorticoids, cromolyn, decongestants, oxymetazoline, naphazoline, phenylephrine *Systemic:* diphenhydramine, dimenhydrinate, tripelennamine, astemizole
Anti-arrhythmics	Adenosine is preferred over verapamil for SVT. Both have been used successfully. Lidocaine is recommended for VT. Electric cardioversion is safe.
Antibiotics	Penicillin, cephalosporin, clindamycin, clotrimazole, erythromycin (not estolate), nitrofurantoin (do not use near term), nystatin
Constipation	Docusate Na^+, calcium, glycerin, sorbitol, lactulose, mineral oil, MgOH
Cough	Diphenhydramine, codeine, dextromethorphan
Diabetes	Insulin, AVOID oral hypoglycemics
Headache	Acetaminophen, codeine, dimenhydrinate, β-blockers (for prophylaxis)
Elevated BP	Labetalol, methyldopa, β-blockers, prazosin, hydralazine
Nausea or Vomiting	Diclectin (doxylamine + pyridoxine), chlorpromazine, metoclopramide (3rd trimester), diphenhydramine, dimenhydrinate, meclizine, cyclizine
Peptic ulcer	Antacids, MgOH⁻, AlOH⁻, $CaCO_3$, ranitidine, sucralfate
Pruritus	*Topical:* moisturizing creams or lotions, aluminum acetate, zinc oxide, calamine lotion, glucocorticoids *Systemic:* hydroxyzine, diphenhydramine, glucocorticoids, astemizole
DVT or PE[1]	Heparin, antifibrinolytic drugs, streptokinase, AVOID warfarin

[1] DVT–deep venous thrombosis; PE–pulmonary embolus *New Engl J Med* 1998; 338: 1128.
[2] Class A: Remote possibility fetal harm, human studies show no fetal risk in 1st trimester.
   Class B: Presumed safety based on animal studies.
   Class C: Teratogenic in animals, no human studies. Class D: Evidence of human risk.

English

Abnormal Vaginal Bleeding in Non-pregnant Women

- *Amenorrhea* - absent bleeding for 6 months
- *Dysfunctional uterine bleeding* - bleeding due to hormonal imbalance
- *Intermenstral* (breakthrough) bleeding - bleeding between regular menstrual cycles - #1 cause = birth control pills use or misuse.
- *Menorrhagia* - menstrual cycles in which bleeding is excessive or prolonged (2/3 of women with menorrhagia will develop iron deficiency anemia)
- *Metrorrhagia* - irregular bleeding at time other than expected period
- *Metromenorrhagia* - prolonged or excessive bleeding at irregular intervals
- *Oligomenorrhea* - uterine bleeding episodes occurring from 35 d to 6 mo

Dysfunctional Uterine Bleeding - DUB

Exogenous steroids (birth control pills) and anovulatory cycles are most common cause. During evaluation, exclude pregnancy and treatable disorders: infection, trauma, bleeding disorders (20% of hospitalized adolescents with DUB - esp. Von Willibrand's disease), endocrine disorders, tumors, fibroids, and cysts. Patients with DUB may have prolonged periods of amenorrhea followed by frequent moderate bleeding or a single episode of profuse painless bleeding.

Classification, Diagnosis, and Management

Class	Hemoglobin	Management [1]
Mild	> 11 g/dl	(1) Iron supplementation, gynecology follow up
Moderate *NOTE:* *High dose* *hormone* *therapy* *may cause* *nausea &* *vomiting*	9-11 g/dl without signs of volume depletion	(1) 4 BCP[2] pills (estrogen/progestin) PO qd until bleeding stops, then taper over 1 week to 1 PO qd **OR** (2) (2) Medroxyprogesterone (*Provera*)[3] 30-40 mg PO qd X 1 week decreasing by 10 mg qd until 10 mg/day, then continue X 3-4 weeks. If bleeding does not stop by 1 week, ↑ to 40-50 mg PO qd, then taper. This agent will NOT protect against pregnancy, use other birth control. (3) nonsteroidals (e.g. ibuprofen 400, 600, or 800 PO tid) may lower prostaglandin E$_2$, + decrease bleeding (4) Iron supplement and gynecology follow-up
Severe *EM Reports* *1996; 219*	< 9 or signs/ symptoms of ↓volume (e.g.↓BP or ↑heart rate)	(1) Fluid, blood, and dilation & curettage as needed (2) Premarin 25 mg IV or PO q 4-6 h until bleeding stops. (max 4 doses) Concurrently, *Enovid* 5 mg PO q 6 h X 1 d, then *Enovid* 5 mg PO qd for 21 day, then no pills for 1 week, then begin low dose BCP[2] for next 3 cycles.

[1] Use caution with administration of listed agents if ≥ 35 or cardiopulmonary disease, as cardiac ischemia, and thromboembolic disease risk is increased with these medicines.

[2] BCP - Birth control pill – estrogen + progestins (e.g.*Lo/Ovral, Ortho-Novum 1/50*)

[3] Alternate regimen - *Provera* 10 mg PO qd, increasing dose 10 mg/day until bleeding stops. Once bleeding controlled, this dose can be maintained for total of 3-4 weeks.

Visual Acuity Screen

96

20/800

873

20/400

2843   O X X   20/200

6 3 8 5 2   X O O   20/100

8 7 4 5 9   O X O   20/70

6 3 9 2 5   X O X   20/50

4 2 8 3 6 5   O X O   20/40

3 7 4 2 5 8   X X O   20/30

9 3 7 8 2 6   X O O   20/25

Hold card in good light 14 inches from eye. Record vision for each eye separately with and without glasses. Presbyopic patients should read through bifocal glasses. Myopic patients should wear glasses only.

Pupil Diameter (mm)

. ② ③ ④ ⑤ ⑥ ⑦ ⑧ ⑨

Common Causes of Red or Inflamed Eye

Feature	Conjunctivitis	Acute iritis	Acute glaucoma	Cornea trauma or infection
Incidence	common	common	uncommon	common
Discharge	moderate-high	none	none	watery,purulent
Vision	normal	sl. blurred	very blurred	usually blurred
Pain	none	moderate	severe	mod/severe
Photophobia	minimal to none	severe	severe, consensual[1]	mild to moderate
Conjunctival injection	diffuse, esp. near fornices	mainly circumcorneal	diffuse or perilimbal	diffuse
Pupil	normal	small	mod dilate/fixed	normal
Light response	normal	poor	none	normal
IOP[2]	normal	normal	elevated	normal
Slit lamp examination	clear anterior chamber	cell and flare reaction	corneal edema, appears steamy	positive flourescein stain
Gram stain	± organisms	negative	negative	± organisms

[1] pain while shining light in unaffected eye, [2]IOP - Intraocular pressure normally is ≤ 20mmHg.

Conversion Chart for Schiotz Tonometer

Tonometer reading	Tonometer load in grams				Tonometer reading	Tonometer load in grams			
	5.5g	7.5g	10g	15g		5.5g	7.5g	10g	15g
	pressure in mmHg					pressure in mmHg			
0.0	42	59	82	128	7.5	11	17	25	43
0.5	38	54	75	118	8.0	10	16	23	40
1.0	35	50	69	109	8.5	9	14	21	38
1.5	32	46	64	101	9.0	89	13	20	35
2.0	29	42	59	94	9.5	8	12	18	32
2.5	27	39	55	88	10.0	7	11	17	30
3.0	24	36	51	81	10.5	7	10	15	27
3.5	22	33	47	76	11	6	9	14	25
4.0	21	30	43	71	11.5	5	8	13	23
4.5	19	28	41	67	12	5	7	12	21
5.0	17	26	37	62	13	4.0	6	10	20
5.5	16	24	34	58	14	3	5	8	15
6.0	15	22	32	54	15	-	4	6	13
6.5	13	20	29	50	17.5	-	-	4	8
7.0	12	18	27	47	20	-	-	-	5

Intraocular pressure (IOP) is falsely ↑ if sticky Schiotz plunger, blinking, accommodation, or looking toward nose. IOP is falsely ↓ with repeated measurements, myopia, anticholinesterase drugs, overhydration and scleral buckle operations.

Acute Narrow Angle Glaucoma

As pupil dilates (e.g. dark room or medication), the angle between the cornea & iris obliterates, blocking aqueous humor resorption with an acute ↑IOP.

Clinical Features	Treatment
• Headache, vomiting, eye pain	• Pilocarpine (2-4%) – 2 drops q 15
• Red eye, perilimbal injection	min X 2 h or until pupilloconstriction
• Conjunctival edema with "flare and	• Pilocarpine 1 drop to unaffected eye
cell" in anterior chamber	• Timolol (_Timoptic_) 0.1% 1 drop
• Mid-dilated, poorly reactive pupil	• Diamox 500 mg IV, IM or PO
• Intraocular pressure is usually > 50	• Mannitol 0.5 - 1g/kg IV
mm Hg	• Laser or surgical iridectomy

Central Retinal Artery Occlusion

Causes	Clinical Features
• Cardiac, carotid, vascular disease	• Sudden painless unilateral ↓ vision
• Hyperviscosity disorders, diabetes,	• Afferent pupillary defect (no direct
sickle cell, birth control pills	reaction to light, + reaction if light
Treatment	shone in contralateral eye)[1]
• Best to start within 2 h (try up to 48h)	• Narrow retinal arterioles
• Globe pressure/massage on 5 sec	• "boxcaring" of retinal arterioles from
and off 5 sec for 5-30 minutes	segmentation of arteriolar blood
• ↑pCO$_2$ by breathing in bag or	• Infarcted retina turns gray
95%O$_2$/5%CO$_2$ mixture	• Cherry red macula due to thin retina
• Paracentesis by ophthalmologist	with clear view of underlying vessels

[1]Marcus Gunn pupil

Iritis -acute inflammation of anterior segment of uvea

	Treatment
Suppurative iritis occurs from infection and _nonsuppurative_ from systemic disease. _Clinical features:_ ↓ vision, perilimbal redness, photophobia (consensual photophobia) and ↑ IOP. Slit lamp reveals cell & flare in anterior chamber.	• IV antibiotics if infectious cause
	• Homatropine 2,5% - 1 drop qid
	• Prednisolone 1% - 1 drop qid
	• Systemic nonsteroidal agents
	• Consult ophthalmologist

Temporal arteritis

History		Examination	
• Mean age (years)	70	• ↓Temporal artery (TA) pulse	46%
• Polymyalgia rheumatica	39%	• Tender temporal artery (TA)	27%
• Headache	68%	• Indurated, red (TA)	23%
• Jaw claudication	45%	• Large artery bruit	21%
• Unilateral vision loss	14%	• Afferent pupillary defect,	-
• Limb claudication	4%	cranial nerve palsies, pale,	
• Eye pain, fever, malaise	-	swollen, optic nerve	-
Diagnosis		_Management_	
• ESR > 50 mm in most cases		• Prednisone 60-80 mg PO q day	
• Artery biopsy (not emergent)		• Ophthalmology consult ± admission	

Mydriatics/Cycloplegics

Drug Trade Name	Duration	Effect[1]	Indication	Comments
Atropine sulfate 0.25-2.0%	2 weeks	M, C	dilation uveitis	anticholinergic, do not use if narrow glaucoma
Cyclopentolate HCl Cyclogel 0.25-2%	24 hours	M, C	dilation e.g. exam	same as atropine
Homatropine 2-5%	10-48hours	M, C	dilation	same as atropine
Phenylephrine HCl Neosynephrine2.5-10%	2-3 hours	M	dilation, no cycloplegia	caution: cardiac disease, glaucoma or hypertension
Scopolamine HBr Hyoscine 0.25%	2-7 days	M, C	strong cycloplegia	same caution above with dizziness, disorientation
Tropacamide Mydriacil 0.5-1%	6 hours	M, C	dilation, cycloplegia	same as atropine, only weak cycloplegia

[1] M - mydriatic (pupillodilation), C - cycloplegia. Usual dose of meds listed is 1 drop qd – tid. Higher doses may be used for specific diseases (e.g. acute angle glaucoma pg 74).

Antimicrobials[1]

Drug (Trade name)	Preparation[2]	Use[3]	Dose
Ciprofloxacin Ciloxan	0.3% solution	G+, G-, ulcers	Conjunctivitis[4]: 1-2 drops q2h X 2d, then q4h X 5d.
Erythromycin Ilotycin	0.5% ointment	G+, Chlamydia	apply q4h until clear X 2 d
Gentamicin sulfate Garamycin/Genoptic	0.3% solution 0.3% ointment	G+ and G-	1-2 drops q 2-4 hX 10 d, apply q3-4h X 7-10d
Neosporin[5]	oint or solution	G+ and G-	1-2 drops q4h X 7-10 days
Norfloxacin Chibroxin	0.3% solution	G+ and G-	1-2 drops qid X 7 d
Ofloxacin Ocuflox	0.3% solution	G+, G-, and ulcers	conjunctivitis: 2 drops q2-4h X 2d, + qid X 5d ulcer: 2 q30 min X 2d, 2 qh X 5 d, 2 qid X 3d
Polysporin[6] Polytrim[7]	ophth. ointment ophth. solution	G+ and G- G+ mostly	apply qid X 7-10 d 1 drop q 3h X 7-10 d
Sulfacetamide Na+ Bleph10/Sulamyd	10-30% solution 10% ointment	G+,G-, no pseudomonas	2 drops q 2-3h X 7-10 d, then apply oint. q3-4h X 7-10 d
Tobramycin Tobrex	0.3% sol'n/oint	G+ and G-	see gentamicin above
Trifluridine Viroptic	1% solution	herpes keratitis	1 drop q 2h (max 9 gtt/d), until epithelialization, then q4h X 7d

[1] Infections other than conjunctivitis/blepharitis require urgent Ophthalmology evaluation.

[2] Most solutions are available in 2.5, 5, or 10 ml bottles, and ointment as 3.5 g tubes.

[3] G+ gram positive, G- gram negatives.

[4] Ulcer treatment: Day 1: 2 drops affected eye q 15 min X 6h, then 2 drops q 30 min. Day 2: 2 drops q h, Day 3-Day 14: 2 drops q 4 h.

[5] neomycin,bacitracin,polymyxin B (PxyB) [6] bacitracin, PxyB, [7] PxyB, trimethoprim

Pelvis and Lower Extremity Trauma

Criteria for Pelvic Radiography Following Blunt Trauma[1]

- Disoriented, Glasgow coma scale < 14
- Intoxication with drugs or alcohol
- Hypotension or gross hematuria
- Lower extremity neurologic deficit
- Femur fracture
- Pain or tenderness of pelvic girdle, symphysis pubis, or iliac spine
- Groin or suprapubic swelling
- Pain, swelling, ecchymosis of medial thigh, genitalia, or lumbosacral area
- Instability of pelvis to anterior-posterior or lateral-medial pressure
- Pain with abduction, adduction, rotation, or flexion of either hip

If all criteria were absent, no patients in either study had a pelvic fracture
Ann Emerg Med 1988; 17: 488; and *J Trauma* 1993; 34: 236.

Ottawa Criteria for Detecting Knee Fractures[1]

- Age > 55 years
- Unable to walk immediately after injury or 4 steps in the ED
- Unable to flex 90°
- Isolated fibular head tenderness
- Isolated patellar tenderness

These criteria detected 100% of clinically significant fractures   *Ann Emerg Med* 1995:405

Diagnostic Maneuvers in Knee Injuries

Injury	Test	Technique
anterior cruciate	Anterior drawer	Bend knee 90° and pull tibia anteriorly. Positive test = excess anterior movement of the tibia (esp. compared to the contralateral side)
	Lachman	Flex knee 20°, pull tibia anteriorly while stabilizing femur. Positive test = excess anterior movement of the tibia.
	Pivot shift	Extend knee, internally rotate tibia, apply lateral valgus stress to knee, then flex knee 20-30°. Positive test = jerk is felt at anterolateral aspect of knee.
posterior cruciate	Posterior drawer	Bend knee 90° and push tibia posteriorly. Positive test = excess movement compared to other side.
collateral ligaments	Varus-valgus	With knee 10-15°, apply varus/valgus stress. Positive test = excess movement compared to other side
meniscus	Apley	Lie prone, bend knee 90°, rotate foot while applying heel pressure. Positive test = knee pain
	McMurray	Hyperflex knee and rotate at foot while palpating joint line. Positive test = click, pain or grinding.

Criteria for Ordering Ankle and Foot
Radiographs Following Blunt Trauma

An ankle x-ray series is only necessary if
there is pain near the malleoli and any of
these findings:

   1. Inability to bear weight both
      immediately and in emergency
      department (four steps)
          or
   2. Bone tenderness at the posterior
      edge or tip of either malleolus

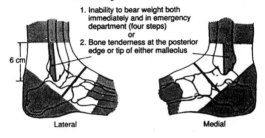

Lateral   Medial

A foot x-ray series is only necessary if
there is pain in the midfoot and any of
these findings:

   1. Inability to bear weight both
      immediately and in emergency
      department (four steps)
          or
   2. Bone tenderness at the navicular
      or the base of the fifth metatarsal

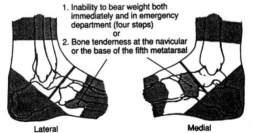

Lateral   Medial

These criteria were found to be 100% sensitive in detecting clinically significant
ankle and foot fractures. Previously criterion of age > 55 years has been invalidated.
Used with permission *Ann Emerg Med*; 21: 383-390.

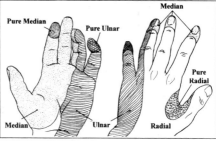

Sensory Innervation of the Hand

Used with permission. Trott . Wounds & lacerations. 1991 Mosby Year Book. St. Louis. MO.186

Nerve	Motor Tests for Nerve Injury
Median	lie dorsum of hand on flat surface, palmar abduct thumb vs. resistance while palpating radial border of the thenar eminence (abd. pollicis brevis)
Ulnar	abduct fingers or pinch paper between thumbs, + prox. index fingers as pull in opposite direction. Nerve injury if thumb IP bends (*Froment's* sign)
Radial	extend fingers and wrist against resistance

Tendons of the Hand

Tendon	Test of Function (Nerves: M-median, R-radial, U-ulnar)
interossei	*dorsal* (spread hand), *volar* (hold paper between fingers) (U
lumbricals	extend wrist + DIP/PIP as fingertips pressed down (M,U)
flexor dig. profundus	flex DIP while MCP and PIP extended (M,U)
flexor dig. superficialis	flex PIP while all other digits extended (M)
flexor dig. superficialis (of index finger)	have thumb + index finger pinch or pick up. If FDS intact, DIP will hyperextend, If not intact, DIP will flex (M)
flex. carpi radialis/ulnaris	flex and radially (M) or ulnar (U) deviate wrist
abd pollicis longus	extension and abduction of thumb (R)
extensor pollicis brevis	extension and abduction of thumb (R)
ext. carpi radialis longus	make fist while extending wrist (R)
ext. carpi radialis brevis	make fist while extending wrist (R)
ext. pollicis longus	lift thumb off flat surface while palm is flat and down (R)
ext. digitorum communis	extension of fingers at MCP joint (R)
ext. indicis proprius	extension of index finger at MCP + other fingers in fist (R)
ext. digiti minimi	extension of small finger while making a fist (R)
ext. carpi ulnaris	extension and ulnar deviation of wrist (R)

dig. - digitorum, flex. - flexor, ext. - extensor, abd. - abductor DIP - distal interphalangeal joint, PIP - proximal interphalangeal joint, MCP - metacarpal phalangeal joint.

Diagnostic Tests for Shoulder Pain

Injury	Test	Technique
Bicipital tend-initis (long head biceps)	*Yergason test*	Flex elbow 90° and pull inferiorly. Grasp elbow with 1 hand, externally rotate arm as patient resists rotation. Positive test = pain with this maneuver.
Rotator cuff injury	*Drop arm test*	Have patient abduct arm while examiner pushes down on forearm. Positive test = arm drops.
Shoulder subluxation	*Apprehension test*	Abduct and externally rotate arm. Positive test = pain and resistance to motion.

Compartment Syndromes

Etiology: ↓ in compartment size (e.g. crush) or ↑ in contents (e.g. swelling, bleed).

Symptoms	Compartment Pressures (CP)	
• Pain (esp. with passive movement)	• Normal	< 10 mm Hg
• Paresthesias (lose vibratory sense 1st)	• Abnormal	10 – 30 mm Hg
• Pallor or Pulselesssness	• Compartment syndrome	30 mm Hg or MAP-CP < 30-40 mm
• Paralysis		

Clinical Features

Compartment	Sensory Loss	Location of Weakness	Passive Movement[1]	Causes Pain at this Location[2]
Interosseous Forearm	None	Finger adduction & abduction	Finger adduction & abduction	Dorsally between metacarpals
Volar Forearm	Volar fingers	Wrist and finger flexion	Wrist and finger extension	Volar forearm
Lateral Forearm	Radial nerve	Wrist and finger flexion	Wrist and finger extension	Lateral forearm
Dorsal Forearm	None	Wrist and finger extension	Wrist and finger extension	Dorsal forearm
Lateral Leg	Top of foot	Foot eversion	Inversion of foot	Lateral lower leg
Anterior Leg	1st web space	Toe extension	Toe flexion	Lateral-anterior tibia
Superficial Posterior Leg	Lateral foot	Plantar flexion of foot	Dorsiflexion of foot	Calf
Deep Posterior Leg	Sole of foot	Toe flexion	Toe extension	Deep calf, medial malleolus, Achilles

Passive movement here (1) causes pain here (2)   *Emerg Med Reports* 1993; 14: 227.

Respiratory Disorders

Predicted PEFR[1] in Adult Females							
Height (in)	**58**	**60**	**62**	**64**	**66**	**68**	**70**
Age (yr) 20	357	372	387	402	417	432	446
25	350	365	379	394	409	424	439
30	342	357	372	387	402	417	431
35	335	350	364	379	394	409	424
40	327	342	357	372	387	402	416
50	312	327	342	357	372	387	401
60	297	312	327	342	357	372	386

[1]PEFR = peak expiratory flow rate. (Liters/min)

Am Rev Resp Dis 1983; 127: 725.

Predicted PEFR[1] in Adult Males							
Height (in)	**63**	**65**	**67**	**69**	**71**	**73**	**75**
Age (yr) 25	492	520	549	578	606	636	664
30	481	510	538	567	596	624	653
35	471	499	528	557	585	614	643
40	460	489	517	546	575	603	632
45	450	478	507	536	564	593	622
50	439	468	496	525	554	582	611
60	418	447	475	504	533	561	590

[1]PEFR = peak expiratory flow rate. (Liters/minute)

Am Rev Resp Dis 1983; 127: 725.

Management Options

General	• Administer O_2 and apply cardiac monitor, pulse oximeter
Inhaled β_2 agonist	• Administer via nebulizer continuous or q30 min if moderate to severe **OR** via MDI 2-4 puffs q 4 hours if mild asthma • albuterol (*Ventolin*) 2.5-5 mg or metaproterenol (*Alupent*) 10-15 mg
Anticholinergics	• ipratropium bromide (*Atrovent*): 0.5 mg in 2.5 ml NS via nebulizer • **OR** 2-8 puffs qid (18 µg /puff)
Steroids	• methylprednisolone (*Solu-Medrol*) 1-2 mg/kg IV **OR** prednisone 1-2 mg/kg PO; continue X 5-7 days (do not taper) • beclomethasone (*Beclovent* or *Vanceril*) 2 puffs tid-qid or 4 puffs bid after stop oral steroids if frequent oral steroids or severe asthma
Other options	• $MgSO_4$ 2 g IV over 15 min if severe asthma and no renal failure • epinephrine 0.3 mg SC **OR** terbutaline 0.25 mg SC q 20 min X 3 • zafirlukast (*Accolate*) 20 mg PO bid 1h pre or 2h post meal; prophylatic
Criteria Predicting Severe Disease & Admission	• Pretreatment PEFR < 80L/min, FEV1 < 1L (25% predicted) • Posttreatment PEFR <200L/min, FEV1 <1.6L (60% predicted) • PEFR ↑< 15% after treatment, pulsus paradoxicus >10 mmHg • Posttreatment PEFR and FEV1 < 60% predicted or PO_2 <60-80, PCO_2 > 40-45, pH <7.35, or SaO_2 <93%

Severity of Asthma Exacerbation (NIH 1997)

Feature	Mild	Moderate	Severe	Pre-Arrest
Breathless	walking	talking	at rest	
Position	can lie down	prefers sitting	sits upright	
Talking	sentences	phrases	words	
Alertness	may be agitated	usually agitated	usually agitated	confused
Respiratory rate	increased	increased	rapid	
Acc. muscles	usually not	common	usually	
Wheeze	end expiratory	all expiration	insp.+expiratory	No wheeze
Pulse	normal	elevated	elevated	$\downarrow$HR
Pulsus para.	< 10 mm Hg	10-20 mm Hg	20-40 mm Hg	$\pm$ absent
PEFR	> 80%	50-80%	< 50%	
PaO_2, (SaO_2)	normal (>95%)	>60mm (91-95%)	< 60mm (< 91%)	
$PaCO_2$	< 42 mm Hg	< 42 mm Hg	$\geq$ 42 mm Hg	

Guidelines for ED Management of Asthma NIH. *Ann Emerg Med* 1998; 31: 579.

History, examination, O_2 saturation, peak flow (PEFR) or FEV1

FEV or PEFR > 50%
- β_2-agonist by MDI or neb. X 3 1st hr
- O_2 to keep sat. $\geq$ 90 %
- Oral steroids if no immediate response

FEV1 or PEFR < 50%
- High dose β_2-agonist + anticholinergic neb q 20 min or continue X 1 hr
- O_2 to keep sat. $\geq$ 90 %
- Oral steroids

Impending arrest
- Intubation + ventilate with 100%
- β_2-agonist + anti-cholinergic neb.
- IV steroids

Repeat exam, PEFR, O_2 saturation as needed

Admit to ICU (see below)

Moderate exacerbation
- PEFR 50-80% of predicted best
- Moderate symptoms
- Inhaled β_2-agonists q 60 minutes
- Oral or increased inhaled steroids
- Treat 1-3 hours, if improvement

Severe exacerbation
- PEFR < 50% of predicted best
- Severe rest symptoms, high risk
- No improvement after initial treatment
- Inhaled β_2-agonists q1h or continuous and inhaled anticholinergics
- O_2 and systemic steroids

Good response
- PEFR $\geq$ 70% X 60 min
- Normal exam

Incomplete response
- PEFR $\geq$ 50%, < 70%
- $\leq$ moderate symptoms

Poor response
- PEFR < 50%, severe
- pCO_2 $\geq$ 42 mm Hg

OR (individualize)

Discharge home
- continue inhaled β_2-agonists + oral steroid
- Patient education regarding medicines, review plan, follow-up

Admit to hospital
- Inhaled β_2-agonist and anticholinergic, O_2
- Oral or IV steroid
- O_2 to keep sat. $\geq$ 90 %
- Follow PEFR,HR,O_2sat

Admit to ICU
- Inhaled β_2-agonist hourly or continuous
- IV steroids, O_2
- Oxygen
- Possible intubation

Prediction of Mortality from Community Acquired Pneumonia

STEP ONE

Is patient > 50 years old	→ YES

↓ NO

Does patient have a history of following? • Neoplastic disease • Congestive heart failure • Cerebrovascular disease • Renal or liver disease	→ YES

↓ NO

Does patient have following exam findings? • Altered level of consciousness (new) • Heart rate ≥ 125 beats/minute • Respiratory rate ≥ 30 breaths/minute • Systolic blood pressure < 90 mm Hg • Temperature < 35°C or ≥ 40°C	→ YES

↓ NO

Patient is in risk category I

> Assign patient to risk classification of II – V *(Step 2 below)*

STEP TWO

Factor	Points	Factor	Points
Male age in years	age	Systolic BP ≤ 90 mmHg	+ 20
Female age in years	age – 10	Temp. < 35°C or ≥ 40°C	+ 15
Live in nursing home	+ 10	Heart rate ≥ 125/minute	+ 10
Neoplastic disease	+ 30	Arterial pH < 7.35	+ 30
Liver disease	+ 20	BUN 30 ≥ mg/dl	+ 20
Congestive heart failure	+ 10	Sodium < 130 mEq/L	+ 20
Cerebrovascular disease	+ 10	Glucose ≥ 250 mg/dl	+ 10
Renal disease	+ 10	Hematocrit < 30 g/dl	+ 10
Altered mentation	+ 20	PaO_2 < 60 mm Hg	+ 10
Respirations ≥ 30/min	+ 20	Pleural effusion	+ 10
		- - -	-

Add Points from	Risk Category	Total Points	30 Day Mortality
Step 2 Above to	Class I	-	0.1 – 0.4%
Determine	Class II	≤ 70	0.6 – 0.9%
Risk Category,	Class III	71 – 90	0.9 – 2.8%
Total Points, and	Class IV	91 – 130	8.5 – 9.3%
30 Day Mortality	Class V	> 130	27.0 – 31.1%

Pneumonia Patient Outcomes Research Team (PORT). *N Engl J Med* 1997; 336: 243.

Pulmonary Embolism (PE)

Pulmonary Emboli Risk Factors	Clinical Features	
• Immobility	• Chest pain	80-90%
• Venous damage (e.g. trauma)	• Pleuritic chest pain	75%
• Hypercoaguability (e.g. cancer,	• Dyspnea	73-84%
prior thromboemboli, nephrotic	• Cough	37-53%
syndrome, inflammatory disease,	• Hemoptysis	13-30%
recent pregnancy (< 3 months),	• Wheezing	9%
estrogen use, sepsis, lupus,	• Respirations ≥ 16/minute	92%
coagulation disorders	• Respirations ≥ 20/minute	70%
• No risk factors in 15% overall	• Rales	51%
• No risk factors in 28% of patients	• Tachycardia	40%
< 40 years old	• Fever > 100° F	43%
	• Calf swelling	30%

EM Reports 1996; 119; *Am J Med* 1977; 358.

Diagnostic Studies	EKG Findings	
• CXR – abnormal in 60-84%	• Nonspecific ST-T changes	50%
• Arterial blood gas–92%↑A-a gradient[1]	• T wave inversion	42%
• Ventilation perfusion scan V/Q – below	• New right bundle branch	15%
• D-Dimer– 95% sensitive,~50% specific	• S in 1,Q in 3, T in 3	12%
• Angiography - > 98% sensitive/specific	• Right axis deviation	7%
• Echo – detects 90% causing ↓BP	• Shift in transition to V5	7%
• CT - ~ 90% sensitive for central PE	• Right ventricle hypertrophy	6%
• MRI – > 90% sensitive for PE	• P pulmonale	6%

A-a gradient: 150 – (paO$_2$ + pCO$_2$/0.8); Normal = patient's age/4 +4.

Emerg Med Reports 1996; 119.

Probability of Pulmonary Embolism

Clinical Suspicion	Ventilation-perfusion Scan Result		
	Low probability[1]	Intermediate	High probability
Low	4%	16%	56%
High	40%	66%	96%

[1]If low prob scan+comorbidity, mortality = 8%. If no comorbidity, mortality = 0.15%.

Emerg Med Reports 1996; 119.

Management of Stable Patients with Suspected Pulmonary Emboli

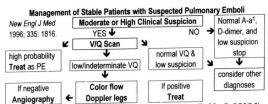

New Engl J Med 1996; 335: 1816.

Moderate or High Clinical Suspicion → YES → V/Q Scan

NO → Normal A-a[1], D-dimer, and low suspicion stop

V/Q Scan → high probability **Treat** as PE

V/Q Scan → low/indeterminate VQ

normal VQ & low suspicion

consider other diagnoses

low/indeterminate VQ → **Color flow Doppler legs**

If negative **Angiography** ←

If positive **Treat**

[1] A-a gradient at sea level: (713) x FiO2 [or 150 on room air]– (PaO2 + PaCO2/0.8)
[1] Normal A-a gradient = age/4 +4

Management Options in Pulmonary Embolism

Heparin	• Load 80 U/kg, drip 18u/kg/hour IV, see page 85.
Thrombolytics	• <u>Indications</u>: shock or significant respiratory distress • <u>Dose</u>: (1) tPA 100 mg IV over 2 hours **OR** (2) streptokinase 250,000 U IV over 30 min, then 100,000 U/hour X 24 hours • May be used up to 2 weeks after symptom onset
Vena Cava filter	• <u>Indications</u>: (1) strong contraindication to anticoagulation **OR** (2) clot develops while adequately anticoagulated
Embolectomy	• <u>Indication</u>: If not anticoagulation candidate & acutely unstable

Management of Suspected Pulmonary Embolism in Pregnancy

There is minimal fetal risk from performing a ventilation-perfusion scan, while an undiagnosed pulmonary embolus can be deadly for both the mother and fetus.

1st Doppler (Duplex) legs	• If abnormal, treat patient. False normal Doppler studies can occur after 20 weeks gestation due to vena cava compression.
2nd perfusion scan	• If Doppler normal, perform reduced dose perfusion scan after IV NS & Foley placed to empty dye from bladder. Normal = no PE.
Ventilation	• Perform ventilation scan if perfusion scan is abnormal.
Treatment	• Use heparin protocol above. *Coumadin* is contraindicated.

Deep Venous Thrombosis (DVT)

Clinical Estimate of the Probability of DVT (total points)[1,2]

Active cancer (or treated past 6 mo)	1	Calf > 3 cm larger than other side[3]	1
Paralysis, paresis, recent leg cast	1	Pitting edema, greater in one leg	1
Entire leg swollen	1	Collateral superficial veins (nonvaricose)	1
Tender along deep venous system	1		
Recent bed-ridden for > 3 days or major surgery within 4 weeks	1	Alternative diagnosis as likely or greater than that of DVT	-2

1 *High* probability (75% DVT prevalence) if score ≥ 3; *Moderate* probability (17% DVT) if score = 1 or 2; *Low* probability (3% DVT) if score ≤ 0.
2 Score is not useful if prior thromboembolism, suspect pulmonary embolus, pregnancy, or on *Coumadin*.
3 Measure 10 cm below tibial tuberosity.

JAMA 1998; 279: 1094.

Evaluation of Suspected DVT Based on Pretest Probability (PTP)- see above

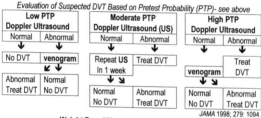

JAMA 1998; 279: 1094.

Weight Based Nomogram for Dosing Heparin

Heparin 80 U/kg IV, then 18 U/kg/hour. Measure PTT q6h. Adjust dose as follows:

Measured PTT	Heparin Adjustment
< 35 sec (< 1.2 X control)	80 U/kg bolus, then ↑rate by 4 U/kg/hour
35-45 sec (> 1.2 - 1.5 X control)	40 U/kg bolus, then ↑rate by 2 U/kg/hour
46-70 sec (> 1.5 - 2.3 X control)	No change
71-90 sec (> 2.3 - 3 X control)	↓ rate by 2 U/kg/hour
> 90 sec (> 3 X control)	stop infusion X 1 h, then ↓rate by 3 U/kg/h

N Engl J Med 1996; 335: 1816.

Low Molecular Weight Heparin for DVT

- This regimen is NOT yet FDA approved. Comparable safety (with lower thrombocytopenia) compared to standard unfractionated heparin has been found.
- <u>Regimens</u> - Enoxaparin (*Lovenox*) – 100 U/kg SC bid OR
  - Dalteparin (*Fragmin*) – 100 U/kg SC bid
- Begin either (LMW) heparin regimen in addition to warfarin on same day. INR should be 2.0 - 3.0 for at least two days before discontinuing LMW heparin.
- <u>Contraindications</u> – major bleed risk, poor compliance/follow-up, renal failure.

Mayo Clin Proc 1998; 73: 545; N Engl J Med 1996; 335: 1816.

Seizures and Status Epilepticus

1. Protect airway, administer O_2, start IV, attach cardiac monitor and pulse oxime-ter, and prepare intubation equipment.
2. Perform stat bedside glucose test, send electrolytes and drug levels.
3. Administer D_{50} 1 amp IV if hypoglycemia, and thiamine 100 mg if malnourished.
4. Intravenous drug therapy as per table. If the first drug is unsuccessful, try another agent. If this is unsuccessful, consider general anesthesia.
5. Treat fever and correct sodium, calcium, or magnesium abnormalities.

Intravenous Drug Therapy for Status Epilepticus

	Drug	Dose & route	Maximum rate	Special features
A	lorazepam	0.05-0.15 mg/kg IV	<0.5-1 mg/min	may repeat q5 min x2
	or diazepam	0.2-0.3 mg/kg IV	<1.0 mg/min	may repeat q5 min x2
	or diazepam	0.5 mg/kg PR	--	may repeat dose x1
B	fosphenytoin	15-18 mg/kg IV	<2.0 mg/kg/min	monitor closely
	or phenytoin	15-18 mg/kg IV	<0.5 mg/kg/min	
C	phenobarbital	15-30 mg/kg IV	<1.0 mg/kg/min	monitor closely
D	pentobarbital (coma)	2-10 mg/kg (load)	slow IV	intubation required;
		0.5-3.0 mg/kg/h	< 1 mg/kg min	vasopressors prn
E	midazolam drip	0.1-0.3 mg/kg IV	< 1-2 mg/min	respiratory and blood
		0.05-0.15 mg/kg/h		pressure depression

Surgical Abdominal Disorders

Diagnoses in ED patients > 65 years old with Acute Abdominal Pain (≤ 1 week)

Physicians should have a low threshold for surgical consultation and admission/observation in elderly patients with undiagnosed abdominal pain.

Pain of unknown etiology	23%	Incarcerated hernia	4%
Biliary colic, cholecystitis	12%	Pancreatitis, UTI, volvulus, abscess	
Small bowel obstruction	12%	constipation, medications	Each 2%
Gastritis	8%	Aneurysm, ischemic bowel, hiatal	
Perforated viscus	7%	hernia, herpes zoster,	
Diverticulitis	6%	reducible hernia, myocardial	
Appendicitis	4%	infarction, pulmonary embolus	
Renal colic	4%	colon obstruction	Each < 1%

Ann Emerg Med 1990; 1383.

Appendicitis

Occurs at all ages peaking at 15-30 y. High misdiagnosis in age extremes/women.

Clinical Features				Diagnostic Studies in Appendicitis	
History		Examination			
Abdomen pain	97-100%	Tenderness		In 1st 24 hours, WBC	
Onset of pain		maximal RLQ	90%	count > 11,000/mm^3	20-40%
Periumbilical	67-87%	Diffusely tender	10%	After 24 hours, WBC	
RLQ[1]	9-26%	Rebound	33-55%	count > 11,000/mm^3	70-90%
In ED, pain is		Fever > 101°F	28%	Urinalysis with > 5	
RLQ[1]	75%	Rigidity	12%	WBC or RBC/hpf	15-30%
Diffuse	17-20%	Absent, hypo-		Ultrasound sensitivity	78-94%
Migration[2]	49-61%	or hyperactive		Ultrasound specificity	89-100%
Anorexia	61-92%	bowel sounds	77%	CT scan sensitivity	92-100%
Vomiting	49-64%	Rectal tender	30-53%	CT scan specificity	> 95%

[1]RLQ – right lower quadrant, [2]Migration of pain from central area to right lower quadrant

MANTRELS Score for Diagnosis of Appendicitis

Total	Action
≥ 7	Candidates for surgery
4-6	Serial exams or further testing is needed (e.g. CT or US)
< 4	Extremely low probability of appendicitis, rare cases have been < 4

Item	Score
Migration of pain to RLQ	1
Anorexia or acetone in urine	1
Nausea with vomiting	1
Tenderness in right low quadrant	2
Rebound tenderness	1
Elevated temperature > 100.4 F	1
Leukocytosis; WBC > 10,500	2
Shift of WBC's; >75% neutrophils	1

A score ≥ 7 is highly suggestive of appendicitis. Nearly all patients have scores ≥ 5.

Resident Staff Phys 1995; 11-18.

Biliary Tract Disease (Biliary Colic)

Risk factors include family, age, females, obesity, weight loss, fasting, cystic fibrosis, malabsorption, medicines (esp. oral contraceptives and clofibrate).

Clinical Features - Biliary Colic	Management of Biliary Colic
• Pain begins 30-60 min after meal	• Treat pain with nonsteroidal anti-inflammatory agents or narcotics.
• Pain duration < 6-8 hours	
• Absence of fever	• Contrary to popular belief anticholinergics (e.g. Bentyl, atropine) are no more effective than placebo for pain relief.
• WBC < 11,000 cells/mm^3 in most	
• Normal liver function tests in 98%	
• Absence of pancreatitis	
• US is >98% sensitive for gallstones	• Surgery follow up

Ann Emerg Med 1996; 28: 273,& 278. Ann Emerg Med 1993; 22: 1363.

Biliary Tract Disease (Acute Cholecystitis)

Clinical Features - Acute Cholecystitis		Management of Acute Cholecystitis
Pain duration > 6-8 hours	> 90%	• Exclude complications by US or CT
Temperature ≥ 100.4° F	25%	(e.g. choledocholithiasis, acute
Murphy's sign	> 95%	pancreatitis, gallstone ileus)
WBC > 11,000 cells/mm³	65%	• Treat pain
Elevated liver function tests	55%	• Administer antibiotics (page 59)
Pancreatitis	15%	• IV NS and take nothing by mouth
Ultrasound sensitivity	85%	• Surgery consult

Ann Emerg Med 1996; 28: 273,& 278. Ann Emerg Med 1993; 22: 1363.

Mesenteric Ischemia

Causes: arterial embolus in 25-50% (esp. to superior mesenteric artery), arterial thrombosis 12-25%, venous thrombosis (esp. coagulopathy) + low cardiac output.
Risk factors: age, vascular/valvular disease, dysrhythmias, congestive heart failure, recent MI, hypovolemia, diuretics, β blockers or vasoconstrictors (e.g. digoxin).

Clinical Features		Diagnostic Studies	
• Abdominal pain	80-90%	• Elevated lactate	70-90%
• Sudden onset pain	60%	• WBC > 15,000 cells/mm³	60-75%
• Vomiting	75%	• Elevated LDH	70%
• Diarrhea (often heme +)	40%	• Elevated CK	63%
• Gross GI bleeding	25%	• Elevated phosphate	30-65%
• _Early_: ↑pain with minimal abdominal tenderness		• Plain xray – obstruction	30%
• _Late_: shock, fever, confusion, distention, rebound, rigidity		• Play xray – thumb printing portal gas, or free air	< 20%
		• CT, & US sensitivity	< 50%
		• Angiography sensitivity	> 95%

Management

• Fluid and blood resuscitation
• Broad spectrum antibiotics (page 59)
• Surgical consult + emergency laparotomy (esp. if bowel necrosis, perforation)
• Mesenteric arteriography will demonstrate thrombosis, emboli, and mesenteric vasoconstriction and allow for selective papaverine administration until symptoms gone or surgery performed.
• Avoid digoxin & vasopressors due to vasoconstriction.

Emerg Med Clin North Am 1996; 571

Pancreatitis

Causes: gallstones, alcohols, drugs (see table), infections (e.g. viral, Mycoplasma, Legionella, Ascaris, Salmonella), trauma, ↑ calcium, high triglycerides and certain metabolic disorders.

Clinical features – Epigastric pain radiating to back ± vomiting. Abdomen may be only mildly tender as pancreas is a retroperitoneal organ.

Complications: ↓Ca^{+2}, ↑glucose, ARDS, renal failure, bowel perforation, sepsis, pseudocyst or abscess formation, bleeding and death.

Select Drugs causing Pancreatitis	
Definite	Probable
azathioprine	acetaminophen
cisplatin, ddl	cimetidine
furosemide	diphenoxylate
l-asparginase	estrogen
tetracycline	indomethacin
thiazides	mefanamic acid
sulfonamides	opiates
pentamidine	valproic acid

Diagnostics - Serum amylase is ↑ in 90-95% with acute pancreatitis. Many diseases cause hyperamylasemia (e.g. salivary gland disorders, abdominal disorders, renal failure, pregnancy, burns DKA, pneumonia). If amylase is ≥ 2-3 X normal, specificity for pancreatitis is >95%. ↑lipase is more specific than hyperamylasemia.

Prognostic Signs in Pancreatitis[1]	
On admission[1]	In 48 hours[1]
Age > 55 y (70 y)	hematocrit fall > 10%
WBC > 16,000 (18k)	BUN rise > 5 mg/dl (>2)
glu > 200 mg/dl (220)	calcium < 8 mg/dl
LDH > 350 IU/L (400)	PaO_2 < 60 mm Hg
AST > 250 U/L	base deficit > 4mEq/L (>5)
	fluid sequestration > 6L(>4)

Mortality: < 1% if < 3, 25% if 3 or 4, 40% if 5 or 6, and 100% if > 6 prognostic signs listed above.
[1]Criteria for gallstone pancreatitis in parentheses

Computed Tomography Grading of Acute Pancreatitis

Grade	CT Findings	Abscess[1]	Mortality
A	Normal CT examination	0%	0%
B	Pancreatic enlargement alone	0%	0%
C	Inflammation of pancreas and peripancreatic fat	12%	0%
D	One peripancreatic fluid collection	17%	8%
E	≥ 2 peripancreatic fluid collections	61%	17%

[1]Rate of abscess formation   *Ann Surg* 1985;201:656; *N Engl J Med* 1994;330:1198.

Diagnostic Studies	Management
• Suspect abscess, hemorrhage, or pseudocyst if fever, persistent ↑ amylase, mass, ↑ bilirubin, ↑ WBC • US - 60-80% sensitive, 95% specific • CT - 90% sensitive, 100% specific • Obtain CT or US if suspect pseudocyst, abscess, gallstones or trauma	• IV fluids and narcotics prn • NG tube if persistent vomiting • If do not improve after 1 week, rule out abscess, pseudocyst, or ascites. • Surgery if: gallstones, bleeding, abscess, pseudocyst > 4 cm, deteriorate despite supportive care

N Engl J Med 1994; 330: 1198.

Toxins that Affect Vitals Signs and Physical Examination

Hypotension			Hypertension
ACE inhibitors	Antidepressants	Nitroprusside	Amphetamines
α & β antagonists	Disulfuram	Opioids	Anticholinergics
Anticholinergics	Ethanol, methanol	Organophosphates	Cocaine, Lead
Arsenic (acutely)	Iron, Isopropanol	Phenothiazines	MAO inhibitors
Ca⁺² channel block	Mercury	Sedatives	Phencyclidine
Clonidine, cyanide	Nitrates	Theophylline	Sympathomimetics

Tachycardia		Bradycardia
Amphetamines	Ethylene glycol, iron	Antidysrhythmics
Anticholinergics	Organophosphates	α agonists, β antagonists
Arsenic (acutely)	Phencyclidine	Ca⁺² channel blockers
Antidepressants	Phenothiazines	Digitalis, opioids
Digitalis, disulfuram	Theophylline	Organophosphates

Tachypnea		Bradypnea	
Ethylene glycol	Salicylates	Barbiturates	Isopropanol
Methanol	Sympathomimetics	Botulism	Opioids
Nicotine	Theophylline	Clonidine	Organophosphates
Organophosphates		Ethanol	Sedatives

Hyperthermia		Hypothermia
Amphetamines	Phencyclidine	Carbon monoxide
Anticholinergics	Phenothiazines	Ethanol
Arsenic (acute)	Salicylates	Hypoglycemic agents
Cocaine	Sedative-hypnotics	Opioids
Antidepressants	Theophylline	Phenothiazines
LSD	Thyroxine	Sedative-hypnotics

Mydriasis (pupillodilation)		Miosis (pupilloconstriction)	
Anticholinergics	Amphetamines	Anticholinesterase	Clonidine
Antihistamines	Cocaine	Opioids	Coma from barbit-
Antidepressants	Sympathomimetics	Nicotine	urates, benzodi-
Anoxia (any cause)	Drug withdrawal	Pilocarpine	azepines, ethanol

Toxins that Cause Seizures

Antidepressants	Cocaine, camphor	INH, Lead, Lithium	Organophosphates
β blockers	Ethanol withdrawal	PCP, theophylline	Sympathomimetics

[1]All agents causing ↓BP, fever, hypoglycemia and CNS bleeding can cause seizures.

Toxidromes

Syndrome	Toxin	Manifestations
anticho-linergic	_Natural_: belladonna alkaloids, atropine, homatropine, amanita muscarina. _Synthetics_: cyclopentolate, dicyclomine, tropicamide, antihistamines, tricyclics, phenothiazines	_Peripheral antimuscarinic_: dry skin, thirst, blurred vision, mydriasis, ↑pulse, ↑BP, red rash, ↑temperature, abdominal distention, urine retention. _Central symptoms_: delirium, ataxia, cardiovascular collapse, seizures
acetyl-cholinesterase inhibition	insecticides (organophosphates, carbamates)	_Muscarinic effects_ (SLUDGE): salivation, lacrimation, urination, defecation, GI upset, emesis. Also ↓or↑ pulse and BP, miosis. _Nicotinic effects_: ↑pulse, muscle fasciculations, weakness, paralysis, ↓respirations, sympathetic stimulation. _Central effects_: anxiety, ataxia, seizure, coma, ↓respirations, cardiovascular collapse
choli-nergic	acetylcholine, betelnut, bethanechol, clitocybe, methacholine, pilocarpine	see _muscarinic_ and _nicotinic_ effects above
extra-pyramidal	haloperidol, phenothiazines	_Parkinsonism_: dysphonia, rigidity, tremor, torticollis, opisthotonis
hemoglo-binopathy	carbon monoxide, methemoglobin	headache, nausea, vomiting, dizziness, coma, seizures, cyanosis, cutaneous bullae, "chocolate" blood with methemoglobinemia
metal fume fever	iron, magnesium, mercury, nickel, zinc, cadmium, copper	chills, fever, muscle pain, headache, fatigue, weakness
narcotic	morphine, dextromethorphan, heroin, fentanyl, meperidine, propoxyphene, codeine, diphenoxylate	CNS depression, miosis (except meperidine), ↓respirations, ↓BP, seizures (with propoxyphene)
sympatho-mimetic	aminophylline, amphetamines, cocaine, ephedrine, caffeine, methylphenidate	CNS excitation, seizures, ↑pulse, ↑BP (↓BP with caffeine)
with-drawal syndromes	alcohol, barbiturates, benzodiazepines, cocaine, narcotics, opioids	diarrhea, mydriasis, piloerection, ↑BP, ↑pulse, insomnia, lacrimation, cramps, yawning, hallucinations

Poisoning Antidotes and Treatments

Toxin	Antidote/Treatment	Other considerations
acetamino-phen	n-acetylcysteine see page 94 for dose	very effective if used within 8h, may be helpful up to 72h
β-blockers	CaCl₂ (10%) 10 ml IV, or gluca-gon 1-2 mg IV/SC/IM	glucagon may help reverse ↓pulse and ↓BP
Ca⁺²channel blockers	CaCl₂ (10%) 10 ml IV, gluca-gon 1-2 mg IV/SC/IM	glucagon may help reverse ↓pulse and ↓BP
cyanide	*Lilly Cyanide Kit* (amyl nitrate, sodium nitrite, and sodium thiosulfate)	Treatment induces methemo-globinemia and ↓BP. Sodium thiocyanate is excreted in urine
digoxin	digoxin Fab fragments	see page 99 for dose
ethylene glycol	fomepizole (*Antizol*) - 1ˢᵗ line ethanol 1 ml/kg of 100% ethanol IV in glucose solution dialysis	15 mg/kg X 1, 10 mg/kg q 12 X 4 ethanol competes for alcohol dehydrogenase, goal is an ethanol level of 0.1 g/dl
isoniazid	pyridoxine up to 25 mg/kg IV	reverses seizures
methanol	ethanol, dialysis (± *Antizol*)	also thiamine and folate
nitrites	methylene blue (0.2 ml/kg of 1% solution IV over 5 min)	consider exchange transfusion if severe methemoglobinemia
opiates	naloxone 0.4-2.0 mg IV	diphenoxylate and propoxyphene may require higher doses
organo-phosphates, carbamates	atropine 0.05 mg/kg IV pralidoxime (PAM)	exceptionally high atropine doses may be necessary; PAM doesn't work for carbamate toxicity
salicylates	dialysis, or sodium bicarbonate 1 mEq/kg IV	goal of alkaline diuresis is serum pH of 7.50-7.55
tricyclic anti-depressants	sodium bicarbonate 1 mEq/kg IV	goal is serum pH of 7.50-7.55 to alter protein binding

Radio-opaque ingestions (CHIPES)	Drugs Cleared by Hemodialysis[1]	
• Chloral hydrate and Chlorinated hydrocarbons • Heavy metals (arsenic, Pb, mercury) • Health food (bone meal, vitamins) • Iodides, iron • Potassium, psychotropics (e.g. phenothiazines, antidepressants) • Enteric coated tabs (KCl, salicylates) • Solvents (chloroform, CCl₄)	• Salicylates • Ethylene glycol • Methanol • Bromide	• Isopropyl alcohol • Chloral hydrate • Lithium
	Drugs cleared by Hemoperfusion[1]	
	• Barbiturates (e.g. phenobarbital) • Theophylline • Phenytoin • Possibly digoxin	

[1] Consult local poison center for more detail concerning latest indications

General Approach to Poisoning

• Treat airway, breathing and BP • Insert IV and apply cardiac monitor • Apply pulse oximeter, administer O_2	• Administer dextrose - 50 ml of D_{50}, naloxone 2 mg IV, and thiamine 100 mg IV

Charcoal

Initial dose is 1 g/kg PO or per NG mixed with cathartic such as sorbitol

Contraindications	Drugs Cleared by Multi-dose Charcoal[1]
• Caustics (acids, alkalis) • Ileus, bowel obstruction • Drugs bound poorly by charcoal (arsenic, bromide, K^+, toxic alcohols, heavy metals [iron, iodide, lithium])	theophylline, phenobarbital, digoxin, dextropropoxyphene, nadolol, phenytoin, diazepam, tricyclic antidepressants, chlorpropamide, nonsteroidals, and salicylates

[1] Administer repeat charcoal doses q 3-4 hours (use cathartic only for 1st dose).

Cathartics[1]

Cathartics theoretically help by ↑ fecal elimination of charcoal-bound toxins, and preventing concretions. Monitor electrolytes closely with their use.

Cathartic choices
• Sorbitol (35-70%) – 1 g/kg PO/NG
• Magnesium citrate 4 ml/kg PO or NG
• Na^+ or $MgSO_4$ – 250 mg/kg PO or NG

[1] Cathartics have never been shown to alter the clinical outcome in acute overdose.

Ipecac

There are no absolute indications for ED use. Ipecac (30 ml PO) delays charcoal administration, incompletely empties the stomach and has many side effects.

Absolute contraindications to ipecac
• Pure caustics or hydrocarbons
• Drugs that cause seizures, ↓mental status, ↓HR, or ↓respirations

Gastric lavage

Directions for Lavage in Overdose	Indications
• Use 36-40 French *Ewald* tube • Lavage stomach with 250-300 ml NS or H_2O aliquots until the return is clear • Protect the airway with endotracheal intubation if there is an absent gag reflex, or altered mental status • Monitor the total input and output from the *Ewald* tube	• Dangerous ingestion within 1 hour • Toxins that slow GI transit • Toxins with possible rapid onset seizure, or ↓mental status • Toxins poorly bound by charcoal
	Contraindications
	• Caustics (acids, alkalis), solvents (hydrocarbons), nontoxic ingestions

Whole bowel irrigation

Administration	Indications
• Administer PO or place NG tube	• Iron, zinc, Li, sustained release meds
• Administer polyethylene glycol (*Go-Litely*) at 1-2 L/hour	• Ingested crack vials or drug packets
	Contraindications
• Stop when objects recovered or	• CNS or respiratory depression
• Stop when effluent clear	• Ileus, bowel obstruction, perforation

Acetaminophen Toxicity

Phase	Time after ingestion	Signs and Symptoms
1	30 min to 24 hours	Asymptomatic, or minor GI irritant effects
2	24-72 hours	Relatively asymptomatic, GI symptoms resolve, possible mild elevation of LFT's or renal failure
3	72-96 hours	Hepatic necrosis with potential jaundice, hepatic encephalopathy, coagulopathy, and renal failure
4	4 days - 2 weeks	Resolution of symptoms or death

Acetaminophen

Ingestion of ≥ 140 mg/kg is potentially toxic. Obtain acetaminophen level ≥ 4h after acute ingestion and plot on the Rumack-Matthews nomogram. A 4h level ≥ 140 ug/ml indicates the need for n-acetylcysteine. On nomogram (page 95), levels above dotted line (--------) indicates probable risk, while levels above the bottom solid line (____) indicate possible risk of toxicity. If time from ingestion unknown, obtain level at time 0 and 4 h later to calculate half-life. If the half-life is > 4 h, administer antidote.

Treatment

Decontamination	• Charcoal is indicated only if toxic co-ingestants are present. • Increase *Mucomyst* dose by 20% if charcoal administered.
N-acetylcysteine *Mucomyst*	• Assess toxicity based on nomogram. • If drug level will return in < 8 hours, treatment can be delayed until level known. *Mucomyst* prevents 100% of toxicity if administered < 8 hours from ingestion. If level will return > 8 hours and ≥140 mg/kg ingested, administer 1st dose of *Mucomyst*. *Mucomyst* is definitely useful up to 24 hours after ingestion, with possible utility up to 72 hours. • <u>Dose</u>: 140 mg/kg PO, then 70 mg/kg q4h X 17 doses. • IV *Mucomyst* is used in Europe and not yet FDA approved.

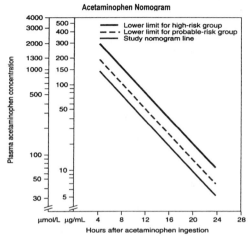

Acetaminophen Nomogram

Used with permission. Rumack BH. *Pediatrics*. 1975; 5: 871.

βeta-Blockers

β1 stimulation - ↑ contraction force + rate, AV node conduction, & renin secretion.
β2 stimulation - blood vessel, bronchi, GI, & GU smooth muscle relaxation.
Propanolol is nonselective, blocking β1 and β2 receptors. Other nonselective β-blockers: nadolol, timolol, pindolol. Selective β1 blockers: metoprolol, atenolol, esmolol, + acebutolol. Pindolol + acebutolol have some β agonist properties.

System	Clinical Features
CNS	• Coma and seizures (esp. with lipid soluble agents – propanolol)
Cardiac	• ↓HR, AV block (1st, 2nd or 3rd), ↑QRS, ↑ T waves, + ST changes • ↑HR with pindolol, practolol, and sotalol. ↓BP is common. • Congestive heart failure can occur.
Pulmonary	• Bronchospasm and respiratory arrest can occur.
Metabolic	• Hypoglycemia is uncommon in adults.

Treatment of β-blocker Toxicity

Option	Recommendations
Gastrointestinal decontamination	• Avoid ipecac. Aspiration & asystole are reported. • Charcoal - repeated doses, ± preceded by gastric lavage
Glucagon	• Indications: ↓HR or BP. Administer 5 mg IV then 1-5 mg/h
Atropine	• Has no effect on BP and will only ↑HR in 25%. • No HR response to 1 mg is diagnostic of β-blocker toxicity. • Administer 0.5 mg IV prn (maximum of 2 mg).
Fluid/pressors	• If ↓BP does not respond to NS, administer α + β agonists (epinephrine/norepinephrine) or pure β agonists (dobutamine)
Other options	• Use pacemaker if no response to above. Consider dialysis if atenolol, nadolol, or acebutolol overdose. • Amrinone – see page 128 for dosing.

Calcium Channel Blockers

System	Clinical Features
CNS	• Lethargy, slurred speech, confusion, coma, seizures, ↓respirations
Cardiac	• ↓HR, ↓BP, AV block (1st, 2nd or 3rd), sinus arrest, asystole
GI	• Nausea, vomiting, ileus, obstruction, bowel ischemia/infarction
Metabolic	• Hyperglycemia (esp. verapamil), lactic acidosis

Treatment

Option	Recommendations
Gastrointestinal decontamination	• Charcoal ± preceded by gastric lavage • Avoid ipecac as aspiration, and rapid ↓mental status occurs • Whole bowel irrigation if sustained-release preparation
Calcium	• Usually ineffective at improving cardiac conduction defects • Primary indication is to reverse hypotension • Administer calcium gluconate 3 g (30 ml of 10% solution) IV over 5 minutes, repeat prn. Alternatively, administer 10-15 mo of calcium chloride 10% IV over 5 minutes.
Glucagon	• Indications: ↓HR or BP. Administer 5 mg IV then 1-5 mg/h
Atropine	• Administer 0.5 mg IV prn symptomatic ↓HR (repeat X 3).
Fluids/pressors	• ↓BP primarily occurs from peripheral vasodilation, therefore administer fluids followed by vasoconstrictors (e.g. norepinephrine, neosynephrine or high dose dopamine).
Other options	• Use pacemaker if no response to calcium, glucagon, atropine.

Carbon Monoxide

Carbon monoxide (CO) exposure can occur from fire, catabolism of heme compounds, cigarettes, pollution, ice-surfacing machines, & methylene chloride (dermally-absorbed paint remover) degradation.

FIO_2	CO half-life
room air	320 min
100% rebreather	80 min
3 ATM hyperbaric O_2	23 min

CO displaces O_2 off Hb shifting O_2-Hb dissociation curve to left. CO also binds cytochrome-A, cardiac and skeletal muscle myoglobin.

Clinical Features

CO-Hb level	Typical symptoms at given level of CO toxicity
0-10%	Usually none, ±↓exercise tolerance, ↑angina, and ↑claudication
10-20%	Frontal headache, dyspnea with exertion
20-30%	Throbbing headache, dyspnea with exertion, ↓concentration
30-40%	Severe headache, vomiting, visual changes
40-50%	Confusion, syncope on exertion, myocardial ischemia
50-60%	Collapse, seizures
> 60-70%	Coma and death
Variable	Cherry red skin, visual field defect, homonymous hemianopsia, papilledema, retinal bleed, hearing changes, pulmonary edema.

- *Delayed neuropsychiatric syndrome:* Certain patients develop permanent neurological or psychiatric abnormalities 3 days to 3 weeks after exposure. There are no reliable predictors of this syndrome, including CO-Hb levels.

Assessment of CO Intoxication

CO-Hb levels	Levels are unreliable & may be low in significant intoxication.
Anion gap	Cyanide and lactic acidosis may contribute to anion gap
Saturation gap	Calculated – directly measured arterial O_2 saturation. This gap also occurs with cyanide, methemoglobin, & sulfhemoglobin.
EKG	May show changes consistent with myocardial ischemia.
Cardiac enzymes	May be elevated from direct myocardial damage.

Treatment of CO toxicity

Criteria for Admission	Criteria for hyperbaric oxygen
• All with CO-Hb > 15-20% • Pregnancy and CO-Hb > 10% • Acidosis, EKG changes, chest pain, abnormal neurologic exam or history of unconsciousness • Persistent symptoms following 100% O_2 X 3 hours	• *Absolute:* cyanide toxic, coma, un-concious > 20 min, abnormal neurological examination, abnormal EKG, arrhythmias, CO-Hb > 25%, pH < 7.20, or neurologic symptoms after 100% O_2 X 3 h • *Relative:* pregnancy, CO-Hb > 20%.

Clonidine

Clonidine is an α-adrenergic agonist with BP lowering properties, and ability to ameliorate opiate withdrawal symptoms. Tablets of clonidine (*Catapres*), in combination with chlorthalidone (*Combipres*), and transdermal patches (*Catapres-TTS*) are available. Used patches may contain up to 2 mg of active drug. Clonidine is rapidly absorbed from GI tract lowering BP within 30-60 min peaking at 2-4 h. Serum half-life is 12 h (6-24 h). Clonidine lowers BP at the presynaptic α_2-agonist receptors resulting in ↓ sympathetic outflow. At high doses, it is a peripheral α-agonist + causes ↑ BP. It is also a CNS depressant.

Clinical Features of Clonidine Toxicity

CNS	• Lethargy, coma, recurrent apnea, miosis, hypotonia
Cardiac	• Sinus bradycardia, hypertension (transient), later hypotension
Other	• Hypothermia and pallor

Treatment

Monitor	• Apply cardiac monitor + pulse oximeter and observe closely for apnea. Apnea often responds to tactile stimulation.
Decontamination	• Charcoal ± gastric lavage. Avoid ipecac.
Atropine	• Indication: bradycardia. Dose: 0.5 mg IV.
Antihypertensives	• Hypertension is transient & usually no treatment is required. If needed, use short acting titratable agent (e.g. *Nipride*).
Fluids/pressors	• Treat hypotension with fluids and dopamine prn.
Naloxone	• 2 mg IV may reverse CNS but not cardiac/BP effects.

Digoxin

Natural sources: foxglove, oleander, lily of the valley, and the skin of toads. Therapeutic range - 0.5-2.0 ng/ml. Severe poisoning may not demonstrate ↑levels.

Clinical Features – Acute Toxicity	
Digoxin level	Usually markedly elevated (obtain > 6 hours after ingestion)
GI and CNS	Nausea, vomiting, diarrhea, headache, confusion, coma
Cardiac	Supraventricular tachycardia, AV blocks, bradyarrhythmias
Metabolic	Hyperkalemia from inhibition of the Na^+/K^+ ATP pump
Clinical Features – Chronic Toxicity	
Digoxin level	May be normal
History	URI symptoms, on diuretics, renal insufficiency, yellow-green halos
Cardiac	Ventricular arrhythmias are more common than with acute toxicity
Metabolic	Potassium low or normal, magnesium is often low

Treatment of Digoxin Toxicity

• Multi-dose charcoal ± lavage.	• ↑K+: page 26. Do not use calcium.
• Atropine 0.5 mg for ↓HR	• Avoid cardioversion if possible (pre-
• Ventricular arrhythmia: lidocaine 1 mg/kg IV ± MgSO₄ 20 mg/kg IV	disposes to ventricular fibrillation).
	• Digoxin Fab fragments (*Digibind*)

Indications for Digibind	Total body load digoxin - TBLD estimates
• Ventricular arrhythmias	TBLD (total body load of digoxin) in milligrams =
• Bradyarrhythmias unresponsive to therapy	• [digoxin level[1] (ng/ml) x 5.6 x weight (kg)]÷1000
• Ingestion of > 0.1 mg/kg	• total mg ingested if digoxin capsules or elixir is ingested
• Digoxin level of > 5 ng/ml	• total mg ingested X 0.8 if another form of digoxin is ingested
• Consider if K+ >5-5.5 mEq/l	

[1] *Chronic ingestions may have normal to mildly elevated digoxin levels.*

Digibind Dosing
• Number of vials to administer = TBLD in mg divided by 0.6
• If ingested quantity unknown consider empiric administration of 10 vials
• One 40 mg *Digibind* vial can bind 0.6 mg of digoxin if amount ingested known
• Dilute *Digibind* to 10 mg/ml & administer IV over 20 min. Serum digoxin levels are useless after *Digibind*, as lab assay measures bound + unbound digoxin. These misleading levels may be exceptionally high, as *Digibind* draws digoxin back into the serum. Once bound, digoxin-Fab complex is renally excreted.

Mushrooms

Treat all toxic mushroom ingestions with IV fluids and GI decontamination. Specific antidotes are useful for certain mushrooms as discussed below. Toxic mushrooms Groups I, II, and VIII (cyclopeptides, monomethylhydrazines, and orellines) cause delayed symptom onset (> 6h from ingestion). Nontoxic ingestions generally cause symptoms < 6 hours after ingestion.

Phases of cyclopeptide mushroom toxicity	Phase	Time	Features
	0	0-6h	asymptomatic latent phase (may last 24h)
	1	6-12h	gastrointestinal phase: vomiting, diarrhea
	2	12-24h	symptoms ↓, ↑liver function tests
	3	>24h	liver failure, shock, renal failure

Clinical Features, Onset, and Treatment of Mushroom Toxicity

Group	Toxin	Onset	Symptoms	Treatment
I Cyclo-peptides	cyclopeptides amatoxins phallatoxins virotoxins	6-10h	See page 99	Multi-dose charcoal, IV NS, ± (penicillin G, cimetidine, thiotic acid, liver transplantation)
II MMH	monomethyl-hydrazine (MMH)	6-10h	CNS-seizures abdominal pain hepatorenal failure	Pyridoxine 25 mg/kg IV or greater, Methylene blue for methemoglobinemia
III Muscarine	muscarine	½ - 2h	Cholinergic	Atropine if ↓ HR
VI Coprine	coprine	½ - 2h	Disulfuram reaction (↑HR, flushed, vomit)	IV fluids
V Ibotinic acid and muscimol	ibotenic acid, muscimol	½ - 2h	GABA effects: (seizures, hal-lucinations), Anticholinergic	Benzodiazepines
VI Psilocybin	psilocybin psilocin	½ - 1h	Hallucinations (~LSD)	Benzodiazepines
VII GI toxins	multiple	½ - 3h	Pain, vomiting, diarrhea	IV fluids
VIIIOrellines	orelline, orellanine	24 - 36h	Renal failure, vomiting	Supportive care, ± dialysis

Insecticides - Organophosphates and Carbamates

Organophosphates irreversibly bind and inhibit cholinesterases at CNS receptors, post-ganglionic parasympathetic nerves (muscarinic effects), and autonomic ganglia and skeletal myoneural junctions (nicotinic effects). Carbamates reversibly bind cholinesterases and are less toxic than organophosphates.

Clinical Features of Insecticide Toxicity

Onset of symptoms	• Usually begin < 24h after exposure. Lipid-soluble organophos-phates (e.g. fenthion) may take days to produce symptoms with persistence for weeks to months and periodic relapses.
CNS	• Cholinergic excess: delirium, confusion, seizures, respiratory depression. Carbamates have less central effects.
Muscarinic	• SLUDGE (salivation, lacrimation, urination, defecation, GI upset, emesis), miosis, bronchoconstriction, bradycardia.
Nicotinic	• Fasciculations, muscle weakness, sympathetic ganglia stimulation (hypertension, tachycardia, pallor, rarely mydriasis)

Organophosphates continued
Diagnostic Studies in Insecticide Poisoning

Labs	• ↑glucose, ↑K⁺, ↑WBC, ↑amylase, glycosuria, proteinuria
EKG	• Early - ↑ in sympathetic tone (tachycardia)
	• Later - extreme parasympathetic tone (sinus bradycardia, AV block, and ↑QT).
Serum *(pseudo)* RBC *(plasma)* Cholinesterase	• Serum levels are more sensitive but less specific than RBC
	• Plasma levels return to normal before RBC levels
	• Mild cases: levels are < 50% of normal
	• Severe cases: levels are < 10% of normal

Treatment

General	• Support airway, breathing and blood pressure. Respiratory depression is the most common cause of death.
	• Medical personnel should gown and glove if dermal exposure.
	• Wash toxin off patient if dermal exposure.
	• Administer charcoal if oral ingestion.
Atropine	• Competitively blocks acetycholine at muscarinic (not nicotinic) receptors. Atropine may reverse CNS effects.
	• <u>Dose</u>: 1-2 mg (or >) q 5 min. Mix 50 mg in 500 ml NS and titrate
	• <u>Goal</u>: titrate to mild anticholinergic signs (dry mouth, secretions) and not to pupil size or heart rate.
	• Treatment failure is most often due to not using enough atropine.
Pralidoxime (2-PAM)	• Reverses nicotinic & central effects, not carbamate toxicity.
	• <u>Dose</u>: 1 g IV over 15 minutes. May repeat q 10-12 hours. Onset of effect is 10-40 minutes after administration.
Atrovent	• Ipratropium bromide 0.5 mg nebulized may dry secretions.

Salicylates

Methylsalicylate (oil of wintergreen) is the most toxic form. Absorption generally is within 1h of ingestion (delays ≥ 6h occur with enteric-coated and viscous preparations. At toxic levels, salicylates are renally metabolized. Alkaline urine promotes excretion. At different acidosis/alkalosis states, measurable salicylate levels change, therefore measure arterial pH at same time as drug level.

Ingestion	Severity	Signs and Symptoms
<150 mg/kg	mild	vomiting, tinnitus, and hyperpnea
150-300 mg/kg	moderate	vomiting, hyperpnea, diaphoresis, and tinnitus
>300 mg/kg	severe	acidosis, altered mental status, seizures, & shock

Clinical Features of Salicylate Toxicity

Direct	• Irritation of GI tract with reports of perforation
Metabolic	• <u>Early</u>: respiratory alkalosis from respiratory center stimulation. • <u>Later</u>: metabolic acidosis - uncoupled oxidative phosphorylation • Hypokalemia, ↑or↓ glucose, ketonuria, and either ↑or↓ Na$^+$
CNS	• <u>Early</u>: tinnitus, deafness, agitation, hyperactivity, • <u>Later</u>: confusion, lethargy, coma, seizure, CNS edema (esp. < 4y)
GI	• Vomiting, gastritis, pylorospasm, ↑ liver enzymes, perforation
Pulmonary	• Noncardiac pulmonary edema (esp. with chronic toxicity)

Indicators of Salicylate Toxicity

Clinical	• Features listed above are associated with toxicity
Ingestion	• Ingestion of > 150 mg/kg may be associated with toxicity
Ferric chloride	• Mix 2 drops FeCl$_3$+ 1 ml urine. Purple = salicylate ingestion
Phenstix	• Dipstick test for urine. Brown indicates salicylate or pheno-thiazine ingestion (not toxicity). Adding 1 drop 20N H$_2$SO$_4$ bleaches out color for phenothiazines but not salicylates.
Salicylate Levels	• A level > 30 mg/dl drawn ≥ 6h after ingestion is toxic • Follow serial levels (q2-3h) until downward trend is established • Arterial pH must be measured at same time, as acidemia increases CNS penetration and toxicity at lower levels. • *Done nomogram* has been proven unreliable
Nontoxic Ingestion	• If none of the following are present, acute toxicity is unlikely (1) < 150 mg/kg ingested, (2) absent clinical features (3) level < 30 mg/dl obtained ≥ 6h after ingestion (unless enteric coated preparation, viscous preparation, or chronic ingestion)

Treatment

General	• Treat dehydration, electrolyte abnormalities. CSF hypoglycemia occurs with normal serum glucose – add D$_5$ or D$_{10}$ to all fluids.
Decontaminate	• Multi-dose charcoal, Whole bowel irrigation (if enteric coated)
Alkalinization	• Add 100 mEq NaHCO$_3$ to 1 L D$_5$NS (20-40 mEq/L K$^+$ if no renal failure. Infuse at 200 ml/hour. <u>Goal</u> – urine pH > 7.5
Hemodialysis	• <u>Indications</u>: renal failure, noncardiogenic pulmonary edema, congestive heart failure, persistent CNS disturbances, deterioration of vital sings, unable to correct acid-base or electrolyte imbalance, salicylate level > 100 mg/dl (acutely)

Chronic Toxicity

Presentation	• Patients are generally older, on chronic salicylates. Neurologic changes and non-cardiogenic pulmonary edema are more common than with acute toxicity. Many are treated for infectious or neurologic disease prior to correct diagnosis.
Drug levels	• Salicylate levels are often normal to therapeutic.
Treatment	• Supportive measures and urinary alkalinization are recommended. Dialyze all with acidosis, confusion, or pulmonary edema regardless of serum level.

Theophylline
Clinical Features

Cardiovascular	• Tachycardia, atrial and ventricular dysrhythmias
Neurological	• Agitation, tremors, seizures
Metabolic	• ↑Glucose, ↑catecholamines, ↓potassium
Gastrointestinal	• Vomiting

Treatment

General	• Monitor for seizures, and arrhythmias. Correct dehydration, hypoxia, and electrolyte imbalances.
Charcoal	• Administer 1g/kg q2-4h. Repeat doses q4h.
Arrhythmias	• β-blockade is preferred for tachyarrhythmias (page 128). Do not use verapamil. It inhibits theophylline metabolism.
Seizures	• Use benzodiazepines (e.g. lorazepam) followed by barbiturates (e.g. phenobarbital). Phenytoin is *contraindicated*.
Hemoperfusion	• Indications (1) seizures, (2) poorly responsive arrhythmias, (3) theophylline level > 100 μg/ml in acute overdose or (4) theophylline level > 60 μg/ml in chronic overdose

TOXIC ALCOHOLS: Ethanol
Ethanol (EtOH) contributes 22 mOsm/L for every 100mg/dl to serum osmolality. The mean elimination rate of ethanol is 20 mg/dl/h (range 16-25)
Brennan Am J Emerg Med 1995; 276.

Clinical Features

CNS	• Euphoria, disinhibition, sedation, Wernicke-Korsakoff syndrome
Cardiac	• ↑HR, ↓BP, atrial (esp. atrial fibrillation) & ventricular arrhythmias
Respiratory	• Aspiration, bradypnea
GI	• Vomiting, bleeding, ulcer, gastritis, hepatitis, pancreatitis
Metabolic	• ↑or↓temperature, ↓glucose, ↓magnesium, ketoacidosis

Alcoholic Ketoacidosis

Due to an ethanol binge in patient who has a decreased caloric intake. Keto-acids, β-hydroxybutyric acid (βHB) and acetoacetate (AcA) accumulate in blood.	*Laboratory values*
	• Anion gap metabolic acidosis
Clinical Features	• Positive Nitroprusside test (serum and urine) detecting acetoacetate
	• Low, normal or mildly ↑glucose
• Vomiting, anorexia, abdominal pain	*Management*
• Hypothermia, dehydration,	• Rehydration (NS or ½ NS)
• ↓HR,↓BP, dehydration,↓urination	• Add D_5 or D_{10} to NS or ½ NS
• Recently terminated alcoholic binge	• Thiamine 100 mg before glucose
• Poor caloric intake X 24-72 hours	• Do not administer bicarbonate

Ethylene Glycol

Ethylene glycol is found in coolants (e.g. automobile anti-freeze), preservatives, lacquers, cosmetics, polishes, and detergents.

Timing	Clinical Features
1-12 hours	• <u>Early</u>: inebriation, ataxia, slurring without ethanol on breath
	• <u>Later</u>: coma, seizures, and death
12-24 hours	• Cardiac deterioration occurs during this phase
	• <u>Early</u>: tachycardia, hypertension, tachypnea
	• <u>Later</u>: congestive heart failure, ARDS, and cardiovascular collapse
	• Myositis occasionally occurs during this phase
24-72 hours	• Nephrotoxicity with calcium oxalate crystal precipitation leading to flank pain, renal failure, and hypocalcemia

Diagnosis	Treatment
• Anion gap acidosis	• Gastric lavage (charcoal is ineffective)
• Osmol gap[2] (measured – calculated osmol) > 10 mOsm/L (page 6)	• $NaHCO_3$ 50 mEq IV to keep pH ~7.40
• Hypocalcemia (EKG - ↑QT interval)	• Ca^{+2} gluconate 10%, 10-20 ml IV if ↓Ca^{+2}, $MgSO_4$ 2g IV over 15 min
• Calcium oxalate crystals in urine	• Pyridoxine & thiamine, each 100 mg IV
• ↑BUN and creatinine	• Fomepizole[1] (*Antizol*) – 15 mg/kg IV, + 10 mg/kg q12h X 4, then ↑ to 15 mg/kg IV q12h until level < 20 mg/dl.
• Serum ethylene glycol level > 20 mg/dl is toxic	
• Serious toxicity has been reported in the <u>absence</u> of anion gap/crystalluria	• Dialysis if (1) oliguria/anuria, (2) severe acidosis, or (3) level > 50 mg/dl (> 20 mg/dl if fomepizole not used)

[1] Administer slow IV over 15 min. If unavailable, load IV ethanol (see Methanol).

[2] Osmol gap may be normal in significant toxicity.

Isopropanol

Isopropanol sources: rubbing alcohol, skin and hair products, jewelry cleaners, paint thinners, and antifreeze. Toxicity occurs after ingestion, inhalation, or dermal exposure (e.g. sponge bath).

Clinical Features	Diagnosis
• Onset of symptoms within 1 hour • Inebriation, CNS depression, coma • Hypotension - peripheral vasodilation • Abdominal pain, vomiting, ↓glucose • Hemorrhagic gastritis, renal failure • Hemolysis, rhabdomyolysis	• Osmol gap (see page 6) • Acetonemia (ketonemia), acetonuria • Mild acidosis (anion gap often absent) • Isopropanol > 50 mg/dl – mild intoxication, > 150 mg/dl – severe • ↓ or ↔ glucose, ↑BUN & creatinine
Treatment	
• Gastric lavage if ingestion < 2 hours. Do not use charcoal (it is ineffective). • Supportive care (maintaining BP and respirations) is all that is required. • Consider hemodialysis if (1) hypotension refractory to conventional therapy or (2) predicted peak level > 400 mg/dl.	

Methanol

Methyl alcohol sources: wood alcohol, solvents, paint removers, shellacs, windshield washing fluids, and antifreeze. Toxicity is from formaldehyde/formic acid. Death has been reported after ingestion of 15 ml of 40% solution.

Clinical Features		Treatment
0-12 hours	• Inebriation, drowsiness • Asymptomatic period	• Gastric lavage (charcoal is ineffective) • NaHCO₃ 50 mEq IV to keep pH > 7.35
12-36 hours	• Vomiting, hyperventilation • Abdominal pain, pancreatitis • Visual blurring, blindness with mydriasis & papilledema • CNS depression	• Folate 50 mg IV q 4 hours • Ethanol (10%) in D₅W – (1) IV loading dose 10 ml/kg, (2) then 1.6 ml/kg/hour (3) dose by 50% if chronic alcohol use, (4) Goal: ethanol level = 100-150 mg/dl
Diagnostic Studies		• Dialyze if (1) visual symptoms, (2) CNS depression, (3) level > 50 mg/dl, (4) severe metabolic acidosis, or (5) history of ingestion of > 30 ml.

• Osmol gap[1] may occur before anion gap acidosis (see page 6)
• Anion gap and lactic acidosis
• Hemoconcentration, hyperglycemia
• Methanol levels > 20 mg/dl are toxic
  (1) CNS symptoms occur > 20 mg/dl
  (2) Visual symptoms occur > 50 mg/dl
		• Stop dialysis and ethanol when methanol levels fall to < 20 mg/dl
		• Fomepizole (*Antizol*) – ± effective but not well studied (see ethylene glycol)

[1] Osmol gap may be normal in significant toxicity.

Tricyclic Antidepressants (TCA)

Clinical features are due to:	ECG findings in TCA overdose
• α adrenergic blockade ($\downarrow$BP),	• Sinus tachycardia
• Anti-cholinergic effects (altered mental status, seizures, $\uparrow$HR, mydriasis),	• $\uparrow$QRS > 100 ms[1], $\uparrow$PR interval, $\uparrow$QT interval, BBB[2] (esp. right BBB)
• Inhibition of norepinephrine uptake (increasing catecholamines)	• Right axis deviation of the terminal 40 ms of the QRS > 120 degrees
• Na$^+$ channel block (causing quinidine like depressive effect on the heart)	• AV conduction blocks (all degrees)
[1]ms – milliseconds; [2]bundle branch block	• Ventricular fibrillation or tachycardia (only occur in 4% who die from TCA's)

Treatment of TCA Toxicity

General	• Apply cardiac monitor, obtain baseline EKG to assess QRS width and QT interval
Decontamination	• Administer charcoal 1 g/kg PO or NG q2-4h. • Consider gastric lavage as anticholinergic effects may slow gastric emptying. • Ensure patent airway & gag reflex prior to decontamination. • Avoid ipecac, as patients may have rapid mental status decline or develop seizures.
NaHCO$_3$	• Indications: (1) acidosis, (2) QRS width > 100 milliseconds, (3) ventricular arrhythmias, or (4) hypotension. • Alkalinization enhances TCA protein binding and reverses Na$^+$ channel blockade and toxic cardiac manifestations. • Dose: 1-2 mEq/kg IV. • Goal: Arterial pH of 7.50-7.55. • NaHCO$_3$ is ineffective for CNS side effects (e.g. seizures).
Fluids/pressors	• Administer 1-2 L NS for hypotension. Repeat 1-2 X. • If fluids are ineffective administer phenylephrine or norepinephrine (not dopamine) due to α-agonist effects.
Anti-seizure medications	• Use lorazepam followed by phenobarbital. • Phenytoin may be ineffective in TCA-induced seizures.
MgSO$_4$	• 25 mg/kg IV may be useful for $\downarrow$ BP, and arrhythmias.
Disposition	*Transfer to a psychiatric facility if all of the following are present:* • no major evidence of toxicity during 6h ED observation • active bowel sounds and $\geq$ 2 charcoal doses are given • there is no evidence of toxic coingestant.

Initial Approach to Trauma Assessment and Management

PRIMARY SURVEY	
Assess **Airway** (*immobilize Cspine*)	• If poor or no air movement, perform chin lift or insert oral or nasal airway. • Intubate if Glasgow coma scale ≤ 8, poor response to above, severe shock, flail chest, or need to hyperventilate. • Cricothyrotomy or laryngeal mask airway if unsuccessful
Assess **Breathing**	• Examine neck and thorax to detect deviated trachea, flail chest, sucking chest wound and breath sounds. • Needle chest for tension pneumothorax, apply occlusive dressing to 3 sides of sucking chest wound, reposition ET tube, or insert chest tubes (36-38 Fr) if needed. • Administer O_2, apply pulse oximeter, measure ET CO_2
Assess **Circulation**	• Apply pressure to external bleeding sites, establish 2 large peripheral IV lines, obtain blood for basic labs and type and crossmatch, administer 2L NS IV prn. • Check pulses, listen for heart sounds, observe neck veins, assess cardiac rhythm & treat cardiac tamponade. • Apply cardiac monitor, obtain BP, HR (pulse quality)
Assess **Disability** (*neurologic status*)	• Measure Glasgow Coma Scale or assess if • **A**lert, or respond to **V**erbal, **P**ainful, **U**nresponsive to pain • Pupil assessment - size, and reactivity
Patient **Exposure**	• Completely undress patient (but keep warm).
RESUSCITATION (Perform simultaneously during primary survey)	
Reassess ABCD's	• Reassess ABCs if patient deteriorates. Address abnormality as identified, place chest tube if needed. • Emergent thoracotomy if > 1,200-1,500 ml of blood from initial chest tube, or > 100-200 ml/h after 1st h. • Administer 2nd 2L NS bolus, then blood prn.
	• Place NG tube + Foley catheter (unless contraindicated).
SECONDARY SURVEY	
History	• Obtain *AMPLE* history (*Allergies, Medications, Past History, Last* meal, and *Events* leading up to injury)
Physical exam	• Perform head to toe examination (including rectal/back).
Xrays	• Obtain cervical spine, chest, pelvic films, CT scans etc.
Address injuries	• Reduce/splint fractures, call consultants as soon as needed, administer analgesics, tetanus, + antibiotics prn.
Disposition	• Initiate transfer, admit, or ready OR. Document all findings, xrays, labs, consultants, and talk to family.

Trauma Score

Respiratory rate	Systolic BP	Respiratory effort	Glasgow coma score
2. ≥ 36/min	4. ≥ 90mmHg	1. Normal	5. GCS 14-15
3. 25-35/min	3. 70-89 mm Hg	0. Shallow	4. GCS 11-13
4. 10-24/min	2. 50-69 mm Hg	0. Retractive	3. GCS 8-10
1. 0-9/min	1. 0-49 mm Hg	*Capillary refill*	2. GCS 5-7
0. None	0. No pulse	2. Normal	1. GCS 3-4
		1. Delayed	
		0. None	

Add points from 5 categories: ≤ 12 needs trauma center, 15-16 has < 1% mortality risk, 13-14 (1-2% risk), 11-12 (2-5% risk), ≤ 10 (> 10% risk). *Ann Emerg Med* 1988; 895.

Glasgow Coma Scale*

Eye opening	Best verbal	Best motor
4. spontaneous	5. oriented, converses	6. obeys
3. to verbal command	4. disoriented, converses	5. localizes pain
2. to pain	3. inappropriate words	4. flexion, withdrawal
1. no response	2. incomprehensible	3. abnormal flexion/decorticate
	1. no response	2. extension/decerebrate
		1. no response

*Total score indicates mild (13-15), moderate (9-12), or severe (≤ 8) head injury.

American College of Surgeons' Classification of Shock

Class	Blood volume lost	Signs and Symptoms[1]
I	< 15% (< 750 ml if 70 kg)	Normal HR, normal vitals, few symptoms
II	15-30% (750-1500 ml)	HR > 100, ↓ pulse pressure, anxiety, UO 20-30 ml/h, capillary refill > 2 sec, RR 20-30
III	30-40% (1500-2000 ml)	HR > 120, ↓ BP, RR 30-40, confused, UO 5-15 ml/h, capillary refill > 2 sec.
IV	> 40% (>2000 ml)	HR > 140, ↓ BP, RR > 35, confused/lethargic, UO - negligible, capillary refill > 3-4 sec.

[1] HR - heart rate, UO - urine output, RR - respiratory rate.

Indications for Cervical Spine Radiographs in Trauma Patients

Absolute Indications	Relative Indications
Midline neck pain - not isolated trapezius	Severe rheumatoid or osteoarthritis
Neck tenderness - midline	Prior cervical fracture
Motor or sensory deficit	Transient motor or sensory symptoms that have resolved[1]
Altered mental status (head trauma, intoxication, drugs etc.)	[1]may indicate herniated disc or transient spinal cord trauma, MRI may be needed
Distracting painful injury	

Cervical Spine Prevertebral Soft Tissue Widths in Normal Adults Mean (mm) ±SD (Range)	Level	Normal Width	Normal range
	C1	8.1 ± 5.8	(3-32)
	C2	5.4 ± 1.6	(2-11)
	C3	5.6 ± 1.6	(2-12)
	C4	9.7 ± 4.4	(4-24)
	C5	14.3±5.8	(2-26)
	C6	14.1±4.4	(3-24)
	C7	13.4±4.5	(3-25)

Prevertebral Widths	Sensitivity[1]
C2 width > 6 mm	59%
C6 width > 22 mm	5%

[1]Sensitivity of C2 width in detecting C1 through C4 fracture and sensitivity of C6 width in detecting C4 through C7 fracture.
Ann Emerg Med 1994; 24: 1119.

Spinal Cord Injury Syndromes[1]

Anterior Cord Syndrome	Central Cord Syndrome
• Flexion or vertical compression injury to anterior cord or spinal artery	• Hyperextension injury
• Complete motor paralysis	• Motor weakness in hands > arms
• Hyperalgesia with preserved touch and proprioception (position sense)	• Legs are unaffected or less affected
	• Variable bladder/sensory dysfunction
• Loss of pain and temperature sense	• Prognosis is generally good and most do not require surgery
• Most likely cord injury to require surgery	
	Brown-Sequard Syndrome
Complete Cord Injury	• Hemisection of cord
• Flaccid below injury level	• Ipsilateral weakness
• Warm skin , ↓BP, ↓HR	• Ipsilateral loss of proprioception
• Sensation may be preserved	• Lose contralateral pain/temperature
• ↓ Sympathetics ± priapism	**Posterior Cord Syndrome**
• Absent deep tendon reflexes (DTR's)	• Pain, tingling, of neck and hands
• If lasts > 24 h will be permanent	• 1/3 have upper extremity weakness
	• Mild form of central cord syndrome

[1] see page 66 for dermatomes, muscles, and reflexes.

Steroid Protocol for Treatment of Acute Spinal Cord Injury

Indications	• Acute spinal cord injury presenting within **8 hours** of injury.
Contra-indications	• Age < 13 y (*controveresial*), nerve root/cauda equina syndrome, gun shot wound, pregnant, steroid use, other life-threatening illness
Protocol	• *Solu-Medrol* 30 mg/kg IV over 15 minutes, then wait 45 minutes
	• If < 3 hours since injury, *Solu-Medrol* 5.4 mg/kg/h over 23 hours
	• If 3-8 hours since injury, *Solu-Medrol* 5.4 mg/kg/h over 47 hours

Bracken. *New Engl J Med* 1990; 322: 1405 & Bracken. *JAMA* 1997; 277: 1597.

Management of Severe Head Injury
(Glasgow Coma Scale ≤ 8)

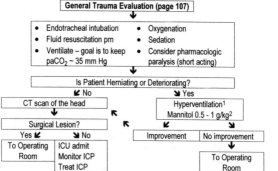

| General Trauma Evaluation (page 107) |

↓

• Endotracheal intubation	• Oxygenation
• Fluid resuscitation prn	• Sedation
• Ventilate – goal is to keep $paCO_2$ ~ 35 mm Hg	• Consider pharmacologic paralysis (short acting)

↓

| Is Patient Herniating or Deteriorating? |

↙ No   ↘ Yes

| CT scan of the head | | Hyperventilation[1] Mannitol 0.5 - 1 g/kg[2] |

↓   ↙   ↘

| Surgical Lesion? | | Improvement | No improvement |

Yes ↙   ↘ No   ↓

| To Operating Room | ICU admit Monitor ICP Treat ICP | | To Operating Room |

[1] Hyperventilation should only be instituted for brief periods if there is an acute neurologic deterioration. A $PaCO_2$ ≤ 35 mm Hg will ↓ cerebral perfusion & can worsen outcome.

[2] Mannitol is only indicated prior to ICP monitoring if signs of herniation or progressive neurologic deterioration occur. Bolus therapy is most effective. Keep serum Osm < 320.

Guidelines for Managing Severe Head Injury.
Am Ass Neuro Surg & Brain Trauma Foundation 1996

Management of Adults with Blunt Abdominal Trauma

Begin Resuscitation - Immediate Bedside Ultrasound

Stable Vitals	**Unstable Vitals**
CT scan (DPL if ? of hollow viscus injury)	DPL 1st unless US shows hemoperitoneum

Liver injury →	Spleen injury →	Surgery if hollow viscus, diaphragm injury Peritoneal sign ± High grade Injuries[1] ± Age > 55-60 > 4-6 U blood 1st 24 hours	**Immediate Surgery** Refractory Low BP Peritoneal signs Diaphragm injury Pneumoperitoneum Positive DPL Cannot assess mental status (controversial)
Grade I - III Observe	Grade I - III Observe		
Grade IV - VI[1] ICU admission Possible surgery	Grade IV - V[1] ICU admit ± surgery		
If Hb falls & stable Angiography & Embolization →	CT in 7 days		
	No success →	Surgery	

Surg Clin North Am 1996; 76: 763.
J Trauma 1998;44:283.

[1] Intraparenchymal rupture with bleed, shattered, avulsion, major vessel injury, > 25% disruption.

Diagnostic Evaluation of Adult Suspected Renal Trauma

Mechanism and Clinical Features

Blunt trauma[1] with pelvic or abdomen trauma, ↓ BP or gross hematuria		**Blunt trauma** with minor mechanism, normal BP and no gross hematuria
CT scan of abdomen/pelvis consider surgery if avulsion, main vessel injury, or shattered kidney		Follow-up urinalysis alone. Consider CT or IVP if persistent or worsening hematuria

Penetrating Trauma

Stable	Possible isolated ureter injury	Unstable
CT scan	CT scan or IVP	One shot IVP in OR

[1] regardless of level of hematuria. *Emerg Med Clin North Am 1998; 16: 145.*

Diagnostic Adjuncts in Blunt Abdominal Trauma

Physical examination: 20% with left lower rib fractures have injured spleen and 10% with right lower rib fractures have injured liver. Nonspecific indicators of liver damage include AST or ALT > 130 IU/L and need for laparotomy includes an arterial blood gas base deficit $\leq$ -6.

Diagnostic tests	Positive Diagnostic Peritoneal Lavage

Diagnostic tests

(1) Computed tomography may miss hollow viscus, pancreatic, mesenteric, and diaphragm injury. It requires hemo-dynamically stability. Oral contrast only aids in picking up < 1% additional pathology on CT, increases aspiration + adds time. (*Ann Emerg Med* 1997; 30:7)

(2) Diagnostic peritoneal lavage (DPL) is more sensitive than CT for identifying need for laparotomy, although it has

Positive Diagnostic Peritoneal Lavage
Aspiration of $\geq$ 10 ml of gross blood
Blunt or penetrating trauma abdomen $\geq$ 100,000 RBC's/ml
$\geq$ 20,000-100,000 RBC's/ml equivocal
Penetrating trauma lower chest $\geq$ 5,000 RBC/ml
White blood cells $\geq$ 500/ml (4h lag)
Lavage amylase $\geq$ 20 IU/L
Lavage alkaline phosphatase $\geq$ 3 IU/L
Bile, food or vegetable matter.

more false positive results and leads to unnecessary laparotomy in many cases.

(3) Ultrasound is less sensitive than DPL in detecting intraperitoneal blood (80-90% vs 98% for DPL), although US detects hemoperitoneum in most patients that require surgery. It is non-invasive, quick, easy to perform and may be repeated frequently.

Penetrating Abdominal Trauma

Indications for Laparotomy

- Unstable vital signs
- Peritoneal signs
- Evidence of diaphragm injury
- Significant GI bleeding

- Bowel protrusion or evisceration
- Impaled or embedded weapon
- Gun shot wound to abdomen[1]
- Positive DPL (see above)

[1]Debate exists as to need for laparotomy in stab wound entering peritoneum.

Penetrating Flank or Back Injuries

Management of such injuries can be difficult as the physical exam is poor at iden-tifying significant intraperitoneal or retroperitoneal injury. Management consists of:

- Immediate celiotomy if shock, or obvious intraperitoneal or vascular injury.
- CT scan with triple contrast (oral, IV, and rectal) if no signs or symptoms of significant injury or gross hematuria alone in a hemodynamically stable patient.
- Angiography may be indicated if retroperitoneal hematoma or retroperitoneal bleeding that is perinephric or near the great vessels.

Trauma - Selected Chest Injuries

Myocardial Contusion

Overview & ED Diagnosis	Features of Myocardial Contusion
The most common injuries are to (1) right ventricle (2) anterior interventricular septum, & (3) anterior apical left ventricle. *Diagnosis*: CXR, EKG, & O_2 saturation on all. CXR findings: pulmonary contusion, 1st or 2nd rib fractures, clavicle or sternal fractures, CHF. EKG findings may take 24 h to develop. Cardiac enzymes are not useful diagnostically.	Car accident speed > 35 mph Steering wheel trauma Anginal chest pain (1-3 d after trauma) unrelieved by nitroglycerin External thoracic trauma (73%) Tachycardia (70%) Friction rub Beck's triad (cardiac tamponade) ↓BP, JVD, ↑HR (< 50%)
Radiologic Studies	*EKG in Myocardial Contusion*
(1) <u>Echocardiography</u> - #1 abnormality is right ventricular wall dyskinesia ± chamber dilation. Echo identifies most problems that require treatment. (2) <u>Radionuclide angiography</u> - assesses ejection fraction (EF). LVEF < 50% or RVEF < 40% are abnormal. (3) <u>Single Photon Emission CT</u> (SPECT) – can detect contusions/ischemia.	Sinus tachycardia 70% Nonspecific ST-T changes 60% Repolarization disturbances 61% Atrial arrhythmias or conduction defects 12% Ventricular dysrhythmias 22% Normal EKG 12% Myocardial infarction 2%

Management
• Consider ICU admission for monitoring if EKG changes, cardiac disease, co-existing trauma or > 45-55 years. Consider echocardiogram or other test (2-3 above), administer O_2 and watch for arrhythmia. • Consider admission for cardiac monitoring if < 45-55 years, nonspecific EKG & no associated trauma. Additional studies are only performed if problems occur. • If < 45 years, normal EKG & ↑ HR resolves, discharge after 1-6 h observation.

Traumatic Thoracic Aortic Rupture

Only 10-20% of patients survive to reach the ED. Rupture most frequently occurs at the fixed immobile ligamentum arteriosum due to a rapid deceleration injury.

Clinical Features	*CXR in Thoracic Aortic Rupture*
• Rapid deceleration injury	• ↑ mediastinal width[1] (52-90%)
• Retrosternal or intra-scapular pain (25%)	• Obscured aortic knob
• Dyspnea, stridor, hoarseness, or dysphagia	• Opacified clear space between aortic knob and pulmonary artery
• Hypotension or hypertension (mean BP 152/98)	• NG rube > 2 cm to the right of the 4th thoracic vertebrate
• Depressed lower extremity BP or lower extremity pulse deficit	• Separation of paratracheal stripe > 5 mm from right lung
• Systolic intrascapular or precordial murmur (31%)	• Left main stem bronchus 40° below horizontal
• Swelling at the base of the neck.	• Left hemothorax/apical pleural cap
• Sternal, scapula or multiple rib fractures	• Multiple rib fractures (esp 1st & 2nd)
• Chest tube with initial output > 750 ml	• NORMAL CXR (up to 15%)

[1] Subjective appearance of mediastinal width (MW) may be more reliable than published measurements. MW on erect PA CXR > 6 cm, on supine AP > 8 cm, > 7.5 at aortic knob or MW at aortic knob/diastoli > 0.25 all correlate with thoracic aortic rupture.

Diagnosis of Thoracic Aortic Rupture

• CXR - misses 6-15% of aortic tears, especially if > 65 years old.

• Aortography - the gold standard test. Perform on all with suspected thoracic aortic rupture. Only delay imaging to repair other life threatening injuries.

• Intraarterial Digital subtraction angiography (IA-DSA) - 100% sensitive in 1 series

• Spiral CT scan is > 90-95% sensitive for aortic rupture. Nearly all patients with rupture have mediastinal hematomas on CT. Some centers are using this modality as a screening tool instead of angiography.

Management of Suspected Thoracic Aortic Rupture

• Perform resuscitation of ABC's as per resuscitation of all trauma patients.

• Diagnosis of thoracic aortic rupture takes priority over all other injuries except life threatening hemoperitoneum and possible brain stem herniation.

• Maintain systolic BP ≤ 120 mm Hg by 1st controlling fluids, sedation, and pain. Use short acting IV agents β-blockade (esmolol + *Nipride*). See page 128.

• Avoid Valsalva (e.g. when inserting NG tube or endotracheal tube).

• Contact thoracic surgeon and prepare for surgery.

Trauma - Penetrating Neck Injuries

Wounds that penetrate the platysma muscle are of major concern. Zone I and III injuries generally require angiography to identify major vascular injury while Zone II injuries generally do not. Information obtained from angiography will generally change the operative strategy in 29% with Zone I and III injuries.

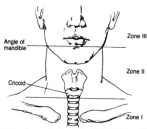

With permission. Tintinalli. *Emergency Medicine.* A comprehensive study guide. 1996 McGraw Hill.

Absolute Indications for Neck Exploration	
Uncontrolled hemorrhage	Stridor or vocal cord paralysis (hoarseness)
Unstable vital signs	Subcutaneous emphysema
Expanding hematoma	Hemoptysis, Hematemesis
Pulse deficits	Neurologic Deficit

Management of Penetrating Neck Trauma	
Airway	• Expanding hematomas, stridor, or other indicators of impending airway compromise mandate endotracheal intubation.
Breathing	• Obtain CXR to exclude pneumothorax. Chest tube prn.
Circulation	• Control bleeding by direct compression and resuscitate with saline and blood if needed. Importantly, complete occlusion of a carotid artery (by compression) for up to 2 hours will generally not cause a neurologic deficit in young healthy patients.
Other Diagnostic Evaluation	• Contact surgical consultants early and exclude cervical spine injury (± xrays), vascular, airway, neurologic, pulmonary and gastrointestinal injury (gastrografin esophogram is diagnostic procedure of choice but has up to a 25% false negative rate).

Urethral and Bladder Trauma

Urethral Trauma

Overview	Retrograde Urethrogram Indications[1]
Pelvic fractures cause most proximal injuries while anterior injuries are usually due to instrumentation, falls, or straddle. Perform abdominal, perineal, & rectal exam, and obtain urethrogram if urethral injury suspected (see table to right).	Penile, vaginal, scrotal trauma
	Perineal trauma
	Blood at urethral meatus
	Abnormal prostate examination
	Suspected pelvis fracture (*controversial*)
	Inability to easily pass Foley catheter
Management	Retrograde Urethrogram Technique[1]
If a partial urethral disruption is identified, a urologist may attempt to carefully (gently) pass a 14-16 F urethral catheter. If unsuccessful or a complete urethral disruption is found, a suprapubic catheter will need to be placed.	Obtain preinjection KUB film
	Place Cooke adapter or Christmas tree adapter on end of 60 ml syringe. (Do not use Foley)
	Inject 10-15 ml of contrast in 60 seconds
	Take xray during last 10 seconds

[1] Use *Hypague* 50%, *Cystografin* 40, or *Renografin* 60, or non-ionic dye (*Omnipaque* or *Isovue*) diluted to ≤ 10% solution with NS.

Bladder Trauma

Overview	Cystogram Indications
All with bladder trauma have pelvic fractures, abdominal trauma requiring CT, or gross hematuria (98%). If gross hematuria or pelvic trauma perform cystogram. Abdominal CT scan can miss this injury. CT abdomen before cystogram so dye does not obscure CT.	Penetrating injury to low abdomen/pelvis
	Blunt abdominal or perineal trauma with (1) gross hematuria, (2) blood at the urethral meatus, (3) pelvic fracture or (4) abnormal retrograde urethrogram or (5) inability to void or minimal urine from Foley catheter
Management	Cystogram Technique
(1) Intraperitoneal bladder rupture will release dye into abdomen, between loops of intestine. Exploration of abdomen + repair is often required. (2) Extraperitoneal bladder rupture shows dye in perivesical tissues, while washout may show dye behind bladder Treat with catheter (Foley if small, suprapubic if large) drainage alone.	After urethrogram, insert Foley catheter
	Obtain baseline KUB
	Instill radiocontrast dye* by gravity until (1) 400 ml or (2) bladder contraction
	Clamp Foley
	Repeat KUB (AP + oblique) , then empty bladder +/- wash out bladder with saline solution
	Then obtain final KUB with oblique film

* Use *Hypague* 50%, *Cystografin* 40, or *Renografin* 60, or non-ionic dye (*Omnipaque* or *Isovue*) diluted to ≤ 10% solution with NS.

Urologic Disorders

The Painful Scrotum

Feature	Torsion of Testicle	Epididymitis & Orchitis	Torsion of Testicular Appendix
Frequency, age 0-20 yr	25-50%	10-25%	30-50%
Frequency, age 20-29	20%	80%	0%
Pain onset	acute onset	gradual onset	gradual onset
Pain location	testis, groin, or abdomen	testes, groin, epididymis	testis or upper pole
Prior similar episodes	often	rare	rare
Fever	rare	up to 1/3	rare
Dysuria	rare	common	rare
Testicle/Scrotum	horizontal high riding testis	firm, red, warm scrotum (>70%)	usually nontender, blue-dot upper testis
Cremasteric reflex	usually absent	may be present	may be present
Pyuria	up to 10%	25-60%	rare
Doppler/Nuclear scan	↓ flow	↑flow	normal flow

Accuracy of Diagnostic Tests for Testicular Torsion in Adults	Test	Sensitivity	Specificity
	Doppler ultrasound	80-90%	80-90%
	Color Doppler US	86-100%	100%
	Nuclear scan	80-90%	>95%

Urology Clin North Am 1996; Radiology Clin North Am 1997;

Management of Suspected Testicular Torsion
- In men under 40 with a painful testicle, assume torsion until proven otherwise.
- Contact a urologist immediately, as early surgical detorsion has the best chance of saving the testicle.
- If the clinical suspicion is low to moderate, consider diagnostic test above after consultation with urologist.
- An attempt to manually detorse the testicle may restore blood flow. To manually detorse, rotate the anterior aspect of the testicle towards the ipsilateral thigh (like opening a book). The testicle will need to be torsed at least 360 degrees. If successful, the patient will experience a marked relief of pain, and the testicle will develop a normal lie (position in scrotum).

$$\text{ug/kg/min} = \frac{16.7 \ \times \ \text{Drug Concentration [mg/ml]} \ \times \ \text{Infusion Rate [ml/h]}}{\text{Weight [kg]}}$$

$$\text{Body surface area (BSA)} = \text{square root of:} \ \frac{\text{height (cm) x weight (kg)}}{3600}$$
$$\text{[in m}^2\text{]}$$

Cardiovascular Drugs: IV Infusions and Mixtures

Drug Solution	1 ml/hr =	Infusion Rate	Drug Preparation
amrinone (*Inocor*)		0.75 mg/kg IV over 2-3 min, then 5.0-10 µg/kg/min IV	100 mg in 100 ml NS
dobutamine (250 mg vial)	1.0 µg/kg/min	5.0-20 µg/kg/min	6.0 mg/kg in D$_5$W in total volume - 100 ml
dopamine (40 mg/ml)	1.0 µg/kg/min	2.0-20 µg/kg/min	6.0 mg/kg in D$_5$W in total volume - 100 ml
epinephrine (1 mg/ml)	0.1 µg/kg/min	0.1-1.0 µg/kg/min	0.6 mg/kg in D$_5$W in total volume 100 ml
esmolol (*Brevibloc*)		500 µg/kg over 1st min, then 50-200 µg/kg/min	5 g in D$_5$W in total volume - 500 ml
fosphenytoin (*Cerebyx*)		100-150 mg/min [loading dose 15-20 mg/kg IV or IM]	500 mg (PE)[1] - 10 ml [1]phenytoin equivalents
isoproterenol (1 mg/5 ml)	0.1 µg/kg/min	0.1-1.0 µg/kg/min	0.6 mg/kg in D$_5$W in total volume - 100 ml
nitroglycerin (*Tridil*)	3.3 µg/min	start 5 µg/min titrate as needed	50 mg in D$_5$W in total volume - 250 ml
norepinephrine (1 mg/ml)	0.1 µg/kg/min	0.1-1.0 µg/kg/min	0.6 mg/kg in D$_5$W in total volume - 100 ml
labetolol (*Normodyne*)		0.25 mg/kg over 2 min, double to 0.5 mg/kg in 10 min, then double to 1 mg/kg in 20 min, MAX 300 mg	200 mg in D$_5$W in total volume - 250 ml
lidocaine 2% (20 mg/ml)	0.13 mg/min	1 mg/kg, may repeat 0.5 mg/kg up to 3 mg/kg,then 1-4mg/min	2g in D$_5$W in total volume - 250 ml
phenylephrine (10 mg/ml)	1.33 µg/min	0.5-5 µg/kg/min	20 mg in D$_5$W in total volume 250 ml
procainamide (100 mg/ml)	20 µg/min	20-80 µg/kg/min	300 mg in D$_5$W in total volume - 250 ml
sodium nitro-prusside (*Nipride*)	3.3 µg/min	0.5-8 µg/kg/min	50 mg in D$_5$W in total volume - 250 ml

Ordering Books From Tarascon Publishing

FAX	PHONE	INTERNET	MAIL
Fax credit card orders 24 hrs/day toll free to **877.929.9926**	For phone orders or customer service, call **800.929.9926**	Internet credit card orders available through our website **www.tarascon.com**	Mail order & check to: **Tarascon Publishing** PO Box 1159 Loma Linda, CA 92354

Name
Address

City	State	Zip

Please send me:	Quantity	Price (table)
Tarascon Pocket Pharmacopoeia • New 1999 edition of the classic drug reference work!		$
Tarascon Internal Med & Critical Care Pocketbk • 1st edition of this acclaimed reference! (released 1997)		$
Tarascon Adult Emergency Pocketbook • New book for 1999! Companion to the peds book!		$
Tarascon Pediatric Emergency Pocketbook • New 1999 3rd edition of this invaluable pocket guide!		$

Price per Copy by Number of Copies Ordered

Number copies ordered	1–9	10–49	50-99	≥100
Pocket Pharmacopoeia	$7.95	$6.95	$5.95	$5.55
Internal Med Pocketbook	$9.95	$8.25	$7.45	$6.95
Adult Emerg Pocketbook	$9.95	$8.25	$7.45	$6.95
Peds Emerg Pocketbook	$9.95	$8.25	$7.45	$6.95

Subtotal	$
In CA only Add 7.75% Sales Tax	$
Shipping & handling (see table)	$
TOTAL	$

Shipping & Handling

If subtotal →	<$10	$10-29	$30-99	$100-500
Standard shipping	$1.00	$2.00	$3.50	$8.00
UPS 2-day air*	$5.00	$8.00	$10.00	$20.00

*No post office boxes

☐ **Charge credit card**: ☐ VISA ☐ Mastercard ☐ American Express

Card number	Exp Date
Signature	Phone